**Searching
Skills Toolkit**

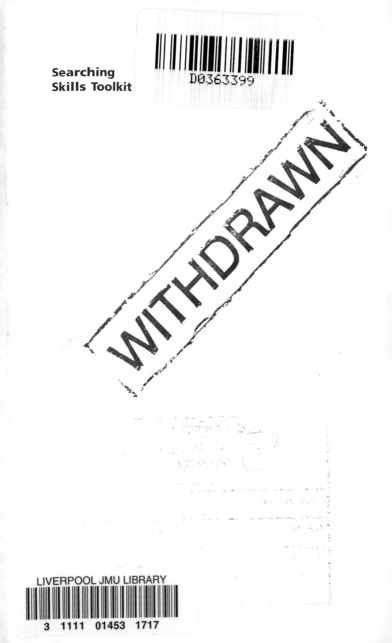

Without the belief of my family and, in particular, my husband, none of this would have been possible.

Caroline De Brún (née Papi).

Searching Skills Toolkit
Finding the Evidence

Second Edition

Caroline De Brún
Clinical Support Librarian
UCL Library Services and Royal Free London NHS Foundation Trust
London, UK

Nicola Pearce-Smith
Information Scientist
Department of Knowledge and Information Science
Summertown Pavilion
Middle Way
Oxford, UK

SERIES EDITORS:

Carl Heneghan
Rafael Perera
Douglas Badenoch

BMJ|Books

WILEY Blackwell

This edition first published 2014 © 2014 by John Wiley & Sons, Ltd.
First Edition published 2009 © 2009 by Caroline De Brún and Nicola Pearce-Smith

BMJ Books is an imprint of BMJ Publishing Group Limited, used under licence by John Wiley & Sons.

Registered office: John Wiley & Sons, Ltd, The Atrium, Southern Gate, Chichester, West Sussex, PO19 8SQ, UK

Editorial offices: 9600 Garsington Road, Oxford, OX4 2DQ, UK
The Atrium, Southern Gate, Chichester, West Sussex, PO19 8SQ, UK
111 River Street, Hoboken, NJ 07030-5774, USA

For details of our global editorial offices, for customer services and for information about how to apply for permission to reuse the copyright material in this book please see our website at www.wiley.com/wiley-blackwell

The right of the authors to be identified as the authors of this work has been asserted in accordance with the UK Copyright, Designs and Patents Act 1988.

The library of Congress Cataloging-in-Publication Data has been applied for
Paperback ISBN: 978-1-118-46313-0

A catalogue record for this book is available from the British Library.

Wiley also publishes its books in a variety of electronic formats. Some content that appears in print may not be available in electronic books.

Cover Design by Andy Meaden.
Cover Images from iStockphoto: Inset 1: (number not known); Inset 2: # 20139828 © Jirsak; Inset 3: #20212066 © ideabug; Inset 4: #3943709 © ChristianNasca.

Set in 7/9 pt Frutiger Light by Toppan Best-set Premedia Limited
Printed and bound in Malaysia by Vivar Printing Sdn Bhd

1 2014

Contents

CHAPTER 1
Introduction

This new edition of the *Searching Skills Toolkit* contains updated instructions and examples for searching a range of healthcare databases, highlighting new features which have evolved as a consequence of technological advances. The sections within some chapters have been reorganised in order to emphasise the steps of the search process and the hierarchy of evidence. There were many web sources included in the first edition, and these have been updated and added to. The chapter on reference management software now includes open source software, such as Mendeley and Zotero, and Appendix 2 on teaching resources contains a new training exercise, for trainers to use in their search skills sessions.

The details in this toolkit are correct at the time of going to press, but please be aware that the Internet is constantly evolving, and the features and appearance of some resources may change slightly as technology progresses. However, the principles and resources underpinning this toolkit are transferable and adaptable to any changes that might arise.

Additionally, this edition contains two new chapters. The first – Chapter 12: Quality improvement and value: sources – focuses on sources of information for health management, quality improvement and cost-effectiveness, to support evidence-based (EB) management decision-making. This chapter is particularly aimed at commissioners, policymakers and health managers. The second new chapter – Chapter 13: Patient information: sources – has been written to help health professionals find good quality health information for patients and their carers. Involvement in the treatment decision-making process is beneficial to the patient and the health service, and is high on government agendas, so it is important that patients have the right information to help them make informed choices that suit them.

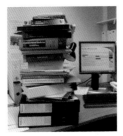

Evidence-based medicine
The concept 'evidence-based medicine' was first used by David Sackett and colleagues at McMaster in Ontario, Canada in the early 1990s. It means

Searching Skills Toolkit: Finding the Evidence, Second Edition. Caroline De Brún and Nicola Pearce-Smith.
© 2014 John Wiley & Sons, Ltd. Published 2014 by John Wiley & Sons, Ltd.

"... the integration of best research evidence with clinical expertise and patient values."[1]

Thus the aim of evidence-based practice (EBP) is to improve the quality of information on which decisions are made.

EBP provides resources to help health professionals find the best quality information to answer their clinical questions. Without these resources, health professionals become overloaded with information, and don't have the time to appraise all the current material published.

In 1972, Archie Cochrane, a British epidemiologist, became concerned that most decisions about interventions were based on an unstructured selection of information, of varying quality.

When making choices at home, such as what car to buy, we usually do some background research, for example, ask friends, look at car magazines, television programmes about cars, etc. We don't have all the answers, not as professionals and not as human beings. We may have gut instincts to guide us, and these can be useful. But you cannot base your choice on gut instinct. Intuition based on professional expertise is part of the evidence-based practice concept, and can be applied to patient care, as long as it is supported by the best available research evidence.

Why search?

Searching skills are a necessity for all health professionals who want to stay up to date with best practice, particularly with the vast increase in research publication and the improved access to research via open access journals. Health professionals need to know how to find and appraise all this research. In 1865, the US National Library of Medicine began indexing medical literature, starting with 1600 references, and reaching 10 million by 2006.[2] In 1999 there was an estimated 32 000 medical journals around the world;[3] the medical literature expands at a rate of 7% per year, doubling approximately every 10–15 years.[4] Currently 400 000 articles are added to the biomedical literature each year.[5]

[1] Sackett, D.L., Strauss, S.E., Richardson, W.S., Rosengerg, W. & Haynes, R.B. 2000. *Evidence-based Medicine: How to Practice and Teach EBM*, Churchill Livingstone, Edinburgh.

[2] Bastian, H., Glasziou, P. & Chalmers, I. 2010. Seventy-Five Trials and Eleven Systematic Reviews a Day: How Will We Ever Keep Up? *PLoS Medicine*, 7(9), e1000326. doi:10.1371/journal.pmed.1000326.

[3] Library and Information Statistics Unit. 1999 Library and Information Statistics Tables, 1998, University of Loughborough, Loughborough.

[4] Price, D.S. 1981. The development and structure of the biomedical literature. In Warren, K.S. Ed. *Coping with the Biomedical Literature: a Primer for the Scientist and Clinicians*. Praeger, Westport, CT, USA.

[5] Davis, D.A., Ciurea, I., Flanagan, T.M. & Perrier, L. 2004. Solving the information overload problem: a letter from Canada. *Medical Journal of Australia*, 180(6 Suppl), S68–S71.

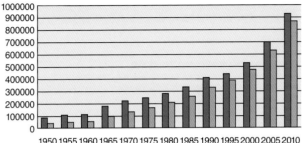

Figure 1.1 Of note, 50 years ago, a greater proportion of the research was published in languages other than English. At the present time, almost 90% of articles are published in English. Data from PubMed, figure created by authors.

Open access resources, such as Biomed Central (www.biomedcentral.com), provide access to 256 peer-reviewed journals covering a range of health-related specialities.

Reading and reviewing all the literature is not feasible for anyone, let alone busy health professionals. There are a range of resources available to help health professionals find the relevant information they require, but some sources contain better quality information and should be targeted first.

Evidence-based practice requires time and a resource investment, as there is so much research to read to inform practice. The aim of this *Searching Skills Toolkit* is to provide you with tools to find the best available evidence faster and more efficiently.

The toolkit has been divided up into chapters covering the basic skills and information you need to know to be an effective searcher. You may wish to work through the chapters in order, but for a quick overview we recommend starting with Chapter 2. This chapter outlines where to go to conduct a health information search depending on how much time you have, what type of publication you require or the specific topic area. A flow chart is included that directs you to search the higher quality evidence first. Where appropriate, references are given pointing you to the essential chapters you need to read, when you see this symbol:

Chapter 9: Refining search results

How do you keep up to date

You can meet your current information needs by a variety of strategies:

- Toss a coin! – May be useful if there are only two options and you already know both.
- Guess – fine if you have the confidence, but what if you're asked to justify your decision?
- 'Do no harm' – don't try anything dangerously innovative!
- Training – remember what you learned during your professional training, which was considered optimum treatment 10 years ago.
- Ask colleagues – but if you ask three people, you may well get three opinions, so who is correct?
- Textbooks – how old are your textbooks and how decayed was the material in them when you bought them?
- Browse journals . . . getting better, but which ones do you choose?
- Literature searching – do you have access to, and the skills to search, bibliographic databases?

Apparently doctors use some 2 million pieces of information to manage patients[6]. Textbooks, journals and other existing information tools are not adequate for answering the questions that arise: textbooks are out of date, and 'the signal-to-noise' ratio of journals is too low for them to be useful in daily practice. When you see a patient, you usually generate at least one question; more questions arise than a doctor seems to recognise. Most questions concern treatment, some are highly complex. Many questions go unanswered, the main reason being lack of time. Some doctors rarely consider the merits of doing a formal electronic search (or of asking a librarian to do a search for them!).

- Write down one healthcare-related problem you recently encountered.
- What was the critical question?
- Did you answer it? If so, how?

Reflect on how you learn and keep up to date. How much time do you spend on each process? Activities usually identified include: attending lectures, conferences or tutorials, reading journals, textbooks or guidelines, clinical practice, small group learning, study groups, searching electronic

---

[6]Smith, R. 1996. What clinical information do doctors need? *BMJ*, 313, 1062.

resources, and speaking to colleagues and specialists. There is no right or wrong way to learn, but it is impossible to keep up to date with all the latest advances. One way to overcome the information overload is to use a push and pull strategy.

The 'push' method is the information we gather from the variety of sources that we receive across a wide spectrum of topics. This could be lectures, seminars, reading journals or magazines. To improve on this technique you should consider reading some pre-appraised source material. An example is the *EBM journal* or *Clinical Evidence*; this will cut down the time you spend reading.

The second method is the 'pull' technique, whereby you keep a record of the questions you formulate using the PICO principle (described in Chapter 5) and then 'pull' information as you need it. *Clinical Evidence* can be used for this sort of information gathering, but the use of a formal literature search would be more useful in obtaining an answer.

Further reading

Akobeng, A.K. 2005. Principles of evidence based medicine. *Arch Dis.Child*, 90(8), 837–840 available from: PM:16040884
✓**Full text:** www.adc.bmj.com/content/90/8/837.full.pdf+html

Dawes, M., Summerskill, W., Glasziou, P., Cartabellotta, A., Martin, J., Hopayian, K., Porzsolt, F., Burls, A. & Osborne, J. 2005. Sicily statement on evidence-based practice. *BMC Med Educ*, 5(1), 1 available from: PM:15634359
✓**Full text:** www.biomedcentral.com/1472-6920/5/1

Glasziou, P. & Haynes, B. 2005. The paths from research to improved health outcomes. *ACP J Club*, 142(2), A8–10 available from: PM:15739973
✓**Full text:** www.ebm.bmj.com/content/10/1/4.2.full

Whiting, P., Martin, RM., Ben-Shlomo, Y., Gunnell, D. & Sterne A.C. 2013. How to apply the results of a research paper on diagnosis to your patient. *Journal of the Royal Society of Medicine Short Reports*, 4(7), 1–9
✓**Full text:** www.shortreports.rsmjournals.com/content/4/1/7.full.pdf+html

Wilton, N.K. & Slim, A.M. 2012. Application of the principles of evidence-based medicine to patient care. *South Med J*, 105(3), 136–143 available from: PM:22392209

CHAPTER 2

Where to start

The hierarchy of evidence

Not all evidence is equal. One way of making sure you find the best quality evidence is to use a 'hierarchy', such as the 4S structure shown in Figure 2.1.

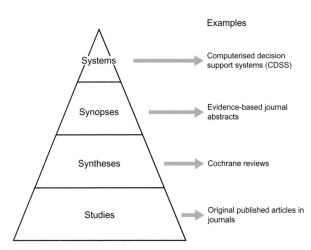

Figure 2.1 The 4S Levels of organisation of evidence from research. Reproduced from Haynes RB,[7] with permission from BMJ Publishing Group Ltd.

Computerised support systems (that integrate and summarise relevant evidence about a patient problem) are developing, and may be more widely available in the future. However, realistically a user will need to look for evidence in the following order:

[7]Haynes, R.B. 2001. Of studies, syntheses, synopses, and systems: the '4S' evolution of services for finding current best evidence. *Evid Based Med*, 6(2), 36–38.

- Synopses – journals containing summaries of evidence with associated commentaries such as *Evidence-Based Medicine*, *ACP Journal Club*, *Clinical Evidence*.
- Syntheses – systematic reviews from the Cochrane Collaboration and the Database of Abstracts of Reviews of Effectiveness (DARE).
- Studies – primary research from journals (randomised controlled trials, cohort studies, case control etc.).

The hierarchy of searching

Use this next chart to help you decide where to start searching. Move through the levels until you have found the evidence you need.

Remember that the quality of evidence is lower the further down the chart you go.

FILTERED SEARCH ENGINES
Clinical search engines, that have been filtered so that only high quality health research is retrieved, for example NICE Evidence Search and the TRIP Database, both of which search a range of evidence-based resources.

GUIDELINES
Guidelines sourced from the UK, where available, such as National Institute for Health and Care Excellence, Scottish Intercollegiate Guidelines Network, Royal Colleges and professional organisations.

SECONDARY RESEARCH
Research summaries from evidence based journals (Synopses), such as Evidence-Based Medicine, and ACP Journal Club, and systematic reviews and meta-analyses (Syntheses) from the Cochrane Library and DARE.

CLINICAL QUERIES
These are special filters, available via PubMed and in the limits of other healthcare databases, which identify evidence to support therapy, diagnosis, aetiology, and prognosis.

HEALTHCARE DATABASES
These can be used for advanced searching, using free-text and Medical Subject Headings. Examples of databases are AMED, BNI, CINAHL, Embase, HMIC, Medline PsycInfo - *(Username & password required)*.

ORGANISATION HOME PAGES
Royal Colleges, professional organisations, academic institutions, NHS organisation homepages.

SEARCH ENGINES
Google, Yahoo, Lycos, Bing, etc.
Use at least 4 and evaluate using DISCERN
www.discern.org.uk

Ask yourself:
1. How much time do I have? For example, 5 minutes or 1 hour?
2. What type of publication am I looking for? For example, guideline or a systematic review?
3. Is my query about a specific topic? For example, drug or safety information, a specific condition, or statistic?

1. How much time do I have?

Quick search <5 mins	Key chapter	Related chapters
1. Secondary sources a. Clinical search engines e.g. www.evidence.nhs.uk www.tripdatabase.com b. Synopses e.g. www.ebm.bmj.com c. Syntheses e.g. www.cochrane.org www.crd.york.ac.uk/CRDWeb/	**Chapter 3:** Clinical information: sources *What is covered?* search examples for EB secondary sources	**Chapter 5:** Formulating clinical questions
2. PubMed Clinical Queries www.pubmed.gov Click on Clinical Queries	**Chapter 9:** Refining search results *What is covered?* search by clinical study type, systematic reviews, specific and sensitive searches	**Chapter 5:** Formulating clinical questions **Chapter 8:** Searching healthcare databases **Appendix 1:** Ten tips for effective searching

Intermediate search <1 hour	Key chapter	Related chapters
1. Secondary sources a. Clinical search engines e.g. www.evidence.nhs.uk www.tripdatabase.com b. Synopses e.g. www.ebm.bmj.com c. Syntheses e.g. www.cochrane.org www.crd.york.ac.uk/ CRDWeb/ d. Clinical guidelines e.g. www.nice.org.uk	**Chapter 3:** Clinical information: sources *What is covered?* search examples for EB secondary sources	**Chapter 5:** Formulating clinical questions

Intermediate search <1 hour	Key chapter	Related chapters
2. PubMed – whole database www.pubmed.gov	**Chapter 8:** Searching healthcare databases	**Chapter 5:** Formulating clinical questions
	What is covered?	**Chapter 6:** Building a search strategy
	a. Search effectively using free text and <u>Me</u>dical <u>S</u>ubject <u>H</u>eading/s (MeSH)	**Chapter 7:** Free text and thesaurus
	b. Combine search terms with Boolean operators	**Chapter 9:** Refining search results
	c. Limit your search	**Appendix 1:** Ten tips for effective searching
	d. View and save results	
	e. Use features of PubMed	
3. Search using at least one other (topic-specific) healthcare database e.g. CINAHL, Embase	**Chapter 8:** Searching healthcare databases	**Chapter 6:** Building a search strategy
		Chapter 7: Free text and thesaurus
	What is covered? How to:	**Chapter 10:** Saving citations
	a. Search effectively using free text and thesaurus	**Appendix 1:** Ten tips for effective searching
	b. Combine search terms with Boolean	
	c. View and save results	

Comprehensive search	Key chapter	Related chapters
1. Secondary sources a. Clinical search engines e.g. www.evidence.nhs.uk www.tripdatabase.com	**Chapter 3:** Clinical information: sources	**Chapter 5:** Formulating clinical questions
b. Synopses e.g. www.ebm.bmj.com	*What is covered?* search examples for EB secondary sources	
c. Syntheses e.g. www.cochrane.org www.crd.york.ac.uk/CRDWeb/		
d. Clinical guidelines e.g. www.nice.org.uk		

(Continued)

Comprehensive search	Key chapter	Related chapters
2. Systematic search using many healthcare databases a. Medline b. CINAHL c. Embase d. PsycINFO	**Chapter 8:** Searching healthcare databases *What is covered?* a. effectively using free text and thesaurus b. Combine search terms with Boolean c. View and save results	**Chapter 3:** Clinical information: sources **Chapter 7:** Free text and thesaurus **Chapter 10:** Saving citations **Appendix 1:** Ten tips for effective searching
3. Citation pearl searching	**Chapter 11:** Citation pearl searching *What is covered?* a. Related Citations in PubMed b. Related Articles in Google Scholar c. Author Search d. Keyword Search e. Snowballing	

2. What type of publication am I looking for?

Many focused clinical questions allow you to see what type of research study you need to answer your question. Many databases provide a 'Clinical Query' option, which uses inbuilt filters to limit your search so that you find only systematic reviews or randomised controlled trials. PubMed Clinical Queries is a good example of this service.

Chapter 9: Refining search results

Internet sources for finding different publication types

Before you start it is important to recognise – just like the wise owl – what type of publication is most appropriate to answer your question; for example, for a therapeutic intervention you should look for a systematic review.

Guidelines: are formal documents, which have been developed by a group of professionals, so that other health professionals know what the best practice is for a procedure. The 'AGREE Instrument' is a tool for appraising guidelines www.agreecollaboration.org/instrument/.

NICE Evidence Search
www.evidence.nhs.uk

**National Guideline
Clearinghouse**
www.guideline.gov/

Systematic reviews: collect and critically appraise all studies on a particular topic, providing a thorough and structured summary of what is known and what is not known. Meta-analysis is a summary of the results. The following are recommended sources for finding systematic reviews.

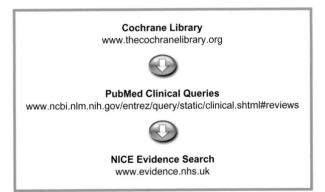

Cochrane Library
www.thecochranelibrary.org

PubMed Clinical Queries
www.ncbi.nlm.nih.gov/entrez/query/static/clinical.shtml#reviews

NICE Evidence Search
www.evidence.nhs.uk

Patient information: Patients and carers need to know where to find the best information available to them. When using health information from Internet sources which have not been validated, use Discern www.discern.org.uk, an online checklist for people to use to help them evaluate the quality of a site. The tool contains a list of questions to ask when looking at a site.

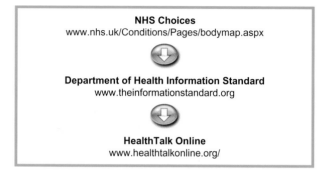

NHS Choices
www.nhs.uk/Conditions/Pages/bodymap.aspx

Department of Health Information Standard
www.theinformationstandard.org

HealthTalk Online
www.healthtalkonline.org/

Randomised Controlled Trials (RCTs): A particular type of study which tests the effectiveness of treatments within a specific patient population who have been randomly allocated to the treatment. The following are recommended sources for finding RCTs.

Cochrane Library CENTRAL
www.thecochranelibrary.com

PubMed Clinical Queries
www.ncbi.nlm.nih.gov/pubmed/clinical

Clinical databases
AMED, CINAHL, Embase, Medline, PsycInfo

Trial registers
Current Controlled Trials - www.controlled-trials.com/
ClinicalTrials.gov – www.clinicaltrials.gov
International Clinical Trial Registry Platform - www.who.int/ictrp/en/
MRC Clinical Trials Unit - www.ctu.mrc.ac.uk/
National Cancer Institute - www.cancer.gov/clinicaltrials/search

If you are unsure about the publication type best suited to your question, use the hierarchy of searching chart near the beginning of this chapter to help you search for the best available evidence.

3. Is my query about a specific topic?

When searching the World Wide Web, it is important to maintain a list of high quality resources. There are tools for storing and sharing favourite web resources and these are described in Chapter 4: Searching the Internet. Here we have listed some useful sources for common topics such as drug information or health statistics – questions on these topics cannot always be answered by searching for research papers.

Topic	Resource

Drug information	British National Formulary
	    www.bnf.org
	US Food and Drug Administration
	    www.fda.gov/
	Merck manual
	    www.merck.com/mmpe/index.html

Safety information	Medicines and Healthcare Products Regulatory Agency
	    www.mhra.gov.uk/index.htm
	European Medicines Agency
	    www.ema.europa.eu/ema/
	World Health Organization
	    www.who.int/medicines/en/

Subject specific e.g. cancer, diabetes, mental health	NICE Evidence Search* www.evidence.nhs.uk

Health services	National Health Service (NHS)
	    www.nhs.uk
	US Department of Health & Human Services
	    www.hhs.gov/
	World Health Organization
	    www.who.int/en/

(Continued)

Topic	Resource

Health statistics	UK National Statistics
	    www.statistics.gov.uk/
	National Center for Health Statistics
	    www.cdc.gov/nchs/
	WHO Statistical Information System
	    www.who.int/whosis/en/
	by country: www.who.int/countries/en/
	e.g. China: www.who.int/countries/chn/en/

* There are numerous subject specific sites to search. You will find information through charities e.g. British Heart Foundation www.bhf.org.uk/, patient groups e.g. Anticoagulation Europe www.anticoagulationeurope.org/, or through clinician associations e.g. American Health Association www.americanheart.org/.

CHAPTER 3
Clinical information: sources

There are a wide range of clinical information sources available to health professionals and patients – these may be in the form of databases, clinical search engines, professional organisations, networks, libraries etc., and can provide access to research from journal articles (e.g. systematic reviews, randomised controlled trials), books, conference proceedings, reports etc. Many sources will be reliable, but others may contain poorer quality information – some sources may index both good and poor quality information (e.g. Medline). Finding the best evidence requires knowledge of the best quality, most appropriate sources. This section describes where to obtain high quality health information.

Medical libraries
You may want to consider involving a search specialist in some of your searches. For some studies (e.g. systematic reviews), you should consider them as an essential part of the project.

Search specialists can be used for:
- specialist collections – databases, books and journals
- accessing full text articles – sometimes the easiest way to get an article is to email your librarian
- development and undertaking of detailed search protocols in systematic reviews – it is worth considering involving a search specialist from the outset when undertaking a systematic review
- teaching and running workshops on search skills.

The Internet
Many people use the Internet to find information, particularly when they need it quickly. But there are good and bad points associated with finding information this way. Also known as the World Wide Web ('www'), the Internet is a vast collection of reliable and unreliable information, personal opinion, expertise, facts, etc. Particularly with the development of social media, and newer

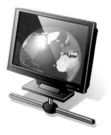

Searching Skills Toolkit: Finding the Evidence, Second Edition. Caroline De Brún and Nicola Pearce-Smith.
© 2014 John Wiley & Sons, Ltd. Published 2014 by John Wiley & Sons, Ltd.

mobile technologies, more information, of varying levels of quality, is being published.

When you search the Internet, try to make sure you are using good quality information sources, or that you use tools to evaluate the quality of the results. Over the next few pages are lists of reliable Internet sources that can be used to find clinical and non-clinical information.

Clinical search engines

These are filtered versions of search engines. They allow you to search information and websites that have met specified criteria, thus retrieving relevant results. Content includes guidelines, systematic reviews, randomised controlled trials, and good quality patient information. Examples of clinical search engines include:

NICE Evidence Search www.evidence.nhs.uk/

NICE Evidence Search is a free web-based portal for staff in the NHS, public health and social care, and is managed by the National Institute for Health and Care Excellence (NICE). NICE Evidence Search provides access to selected, high quality clinical and non-clinical evidence. The content of NICE Evidence Search is subject to assessment before inclusion, to ensure it meets quality criteria.

NHS staff with an Athens password can also get free access to many journals and databases, which are paid for nationally. For more information about the databases and journals available, and how to get an Athens account, click on 'Journals and Databases'.

You can use NICE Evidence Search to search for information using the search box, or you can browse by clinical topic.

Choose a clinical topic by clicking on *A to Z of topics*, then use the categories to see an overview of the evidence on that topic e.g. guidance, commissioning, etc.

My Evidence | Journals and Databases   Sign In

Urinary Tract Infection 🔍

Close ▬

Urinary Tract Infection: Introduction Feedback

A general introduction to Urinary Tract Infection.

Source: Clinical Knowledge Summaries, 25 Jan 2010

Urinary tract infection (UTI) is the name given to an infection of any part of the urinary system.

What is the urinary system?

The urinary system is made up of the kidneys, the ureters (the tubes that carry urine from the kidneys to the bladder), the bladder, and the urethra (the tube that passes from the bladder through the penis, or vulva - which is located between the vaginal opening and the clitoris - through which we urinate).

When we digest food, waste products are left behind in our blood and are removed by either the liver or the kidneys. The most important part of the waste products removed by the kidneys is known as urea. Urea is mixed with water to produce urine. The urine is passed down from the kidneys and into the bladder. Once the bladder is full of urine, the urine is passed from the body, through the urethra, when we urinate.

What is UTI?

A UTI develops when part of the urinary system becomes infected, usually by bacteria. Bacteria can enter the urinary system through the urethra, or more rarely, through the bloodstream. Usually there is no obvious reason why the urinary system gets infected, although some women find that they get UTIs after sexual intercourse.

(vertical tabs at right): Guidance | Commissioning | Information for the public | Ongoing Research | Evidence Uncertainty

Filter by ⍰   Results are currently sorted by relevance (Sort results by: date)   Results 1 - 10 (of 7973) ➕

Areas of interest   Results included for uti
                          Show results for Urinary Tract Infection only
Types of information

Clinical queries   ⊕ CG54 Urinary tract infection in children: full guideline

Sources   ...role of VUR in predisposing to infections..25–28 Although there is...with acute pyelonephritis/upper
                              urinary tract infection can be dangerous for the kidney...between acute pyelonephritis/upper urinary
Medicines and devices   tract infection and cystitis/lower urinary tract infections. 4.7.3 Localising UTI...

Published date   National Institute for Health and Clinical Excellence, 22 August 2007 - Publisher: NICE - Publication type: Full Guidance
                              PDF

Search History   ⊕ CG54 Urinary tract infection in children: NICE guideline

Urinary Tract Infection   ...abnormalities of the urinary tract such as obstruction...clinical guideline 54 – Urinary tract infection in
"integrated care"   ...ren...who have had a lower urinary tract infection should undergo ultrasound...or have had recurrent
Integrated Delivery Of   ...ns. 1.3.1.5 A DMSA...treating symptomatic infections promptly whenever they...clinical guideline
                              ...r tract infection in children 25 VUR...
                              ...Health and Clinical Excellence, 22 August 2007 - Publisher: NICE - Publication type: NICE Guidance

This symbol is an accreditation symbol and recognises the high quality of the material.

Alternatively, use simple search terms to retrieve evidence.

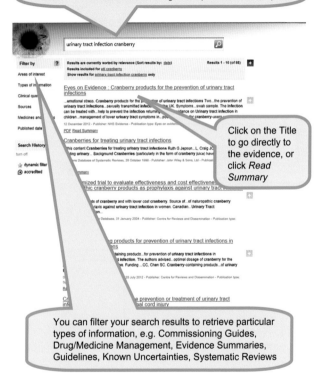

NICE Evidence Search will search for **all** terms entered and lists them in 'relevance' order (based on frequency of terms, quality and date of publication). Use OR if you want to search for alternative terms, e.g. *hemophilia OR haemophilia*

Click on the Title to go directly to the evidence, or click *Read Summary*

You can filter your search results to retrieve particular types of information, e.g. Commissioning Guides, Drug/Medicine Management, Evidence Summaries, Guidelines, Known Uncertainties, Systematic Reviews

TRIP (Turning Research Into Practice) www.tripdatabase.com/
The TRIP Database has three methods of searching: basic search, advanced search, and PICO search, which lets you enter concepts using the PICO (patient/problem/population, intervention, comparison, outcome) framework.

Example: find information on the use of cranberries in the treatment of urinary tract infections.

1. Go to The TRIP Database www.tripdatabase.com/

2. Type in search terms e.g. cranberr* uti. The asterisk means that the database will search for cranberry or cranberries, and uti refers to urinary tract infection.

3. The results will be displayed, together with a breakdown of the results by levels of evidence, starting with evidence-based synopses, followed by systematic reviews, guidelines, clinical Q&A, primary research, and e-textbooks. Videos, images and patient information are also searchable with TRIP.

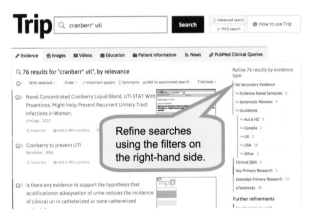

National guidelines

For UK guidance, use NICE Evidence Search at www.evidence.nhs.uk/. Enter search terms and use the filters on the left-hand side to identify guidelines produced by NICE and other national agencies and professional organisations.

International guidelines

These are available from:

- National Institute for Health and Care Excellence (NICE)
  www.nice.org.uk
- Scottish Intercollegiate Guidelines Network (SIGN)
  www.sign.ac.uk/
- US National Guidelines Clearing House
  www.guideline.gov/

- US Agency for Healthcare Research and Quality
    www.ahrq.gov/
- New Zealand Guidelines Group – Guidelines Library
    www.nzgg.org.nz/
- Australian National Health and Medical Research Council
    www.nhmrc.gov.au/guidelines
- WHO programmes and projects
    www.who.int/entity/en/
- British Columbia Guidelines
    www.health.gov.bc.ca/gpac/alphabetical.html
- Institute for Clinical Systems Improvement
    www.icsi.org/guidelines__more/
- Michigan Quality Improvement Consortium Guidelines
    www.mqic.org/guidelines.htm

AGREE is a tool for the purpose of appraising guidelines for research and evaluation: www.apps.who.int/rhl/agreeinstrumentfinal.pdf

Sources containing secondary evidence
Secondary evidence draws together primary research in the form of an overview or structured summary. Forms of secondary evidence include:
- systematic reviews
- critical reviews
- structured abstracts, with or without expert commentaries.

Evidence-based journals
Journals containing informative abstracts with expert commentaries include:
- *Evidence-Based Medicine* www.ebm.bmj.com/
- *Evidence-Based Nursing* www.ebn.bmj.com/
- *Evidence-Based Mental Health* www.ebmh.bmj.com/
- *Evidence-Based Dentistry* www.nature.com/ebd/index.html
- *Evidence-Based Complementary and Alternative Medicine*
    www.ecam.oxfordjournals.org/
- *International Journal of Evidence-Based Healthcare*
    www.blackwellpublishing.com/journal.asp?ref=1744-1595
- *BMJ Clinical Evidence* www.clinicalevidence.com/x/index.html
- *ACP Journal Club* www.acpjc.acponline.org/
These are subscription-based journals, so not accessible to everyone.

The Cochrane Library
Systematic reviews are available via The Cochrane Library at www.thecochranelibrary.com/. The abstracts of Cochrane reviews can also

be browsed and searched from the Cochrane Collaboration site and are available in other languages including French and Spanish.

Example: Find a Cochrane systematic review on the use of cranberries in the treatment of urinary tract disease.
1. Go to The Cochrane Library at www.thecochranelibrary.com/
2. Type in search terms e.g. cranberries uti.
3. Click on the title to access the abstract and, if available, the full text.

DARE
The Database of Abstracts of Reviews of Effectiveness contains structured abstracts and commentaries from the York Centre for Reviews and

Dissemination (CRD) team about other published systematic reviews:
www.crd.york.ac.uk/crdweb/

Online databases

If nothing relevant or up to date is found from the listed sources, then the
next step is to search an online database. These databases contain citations
of journal articles, which have been indexed for easier retrieval. It is
important to remember that the content on most databases will not have
been appraised.

   Because the Medline database is freely available as 'PubMed'
www.pubmed.gov from the National Library of Medicine, we find it useful
in daily searching. The majority of the content is only available in abstract
format, but as open access publishing develops, a growing number of
records are linking to freely available, full-text, research papers, via PMC
www.ncbi.nlm.nih.gov/pmc/ in the USA, UK PMC www.ukpmc.ac.uk/ in the
UK, and PubMed Central www.pubmedcentralcanada.ca/pmcc/ in Canada.

   The following databases are sources of health information to support clinical
and non-clinical decision-making. Bear in mind that the content tends to be
non-appraised research, although peer reviewed and published in professional
journals, and they are therefore better quality than using search engines:

- African Index Medicus *(freely available)*
   www.indexmedicus.afro.who.int/
   African Index Medicus (AIM) collates all biomedical information published
   in or related to Africa.
- AMED *(subscription required)*
   This resource contains abstracts about complementary medicine, palliative
   care, and professions allied to medicine, including physiotherapy,
   occupational therapy, rehabilitation, speech and language therapy, and
   podiatry.
- ASSIA *(subscription required)*
   www.csa.com/factsheets/assia-set-c.php
   This is the Applied Social Sciences Index and Abstracts database, and it
   covers health, social services, psychology, sociology, economics, politics,
   race relations, and education.
- Chinese Medical Collections *(freely available)*
   www.wanfangdata.com/medical/intr.asp
   This resource covers medical journals, dissertations, conference
   proceedings, patents, standards, companies and products.
- CINAHL *(subscription required)*
   CINAHL covers a wide range of topics including nursing, biomedicine,
   health sciences librarianship, alternative/complementary medicine,
   consumer health and 17 allied health disciplines.
- Embase *(subscription required)*
   This is the European version of Medline, containing abstracts of articles on
   medical and pharmacological research.

- Global Health Library *(freely available)*
  www.globalhealthlibrary.net/php/index.php
  This resource contains medical and health documentation from countries, less developed, outside the major industrialised areas.
- Health Business Elite *(subscription required)*
  This is a resource which provides comprehensive journal content detailing all aspects of healthcare administration and other non-clinical aspects of healthcare management.
- Health Systems Evidence *(freely available)*
  www.mcmasterhealthforum.org/healthsystemsevidence-en
  This database has been pulled together by McMaster University, and contains evidence for making decisions about strengthening or reforming health systems or cost-effective programmes, services and drugs.
- HMIC *(subscription required)*
  This database brings together the bibliographic database of two UK health and social care management organisations: the Department of Health's Library and Information Services (DH-Data) and the King's Fund Information and Library Service.
- Indmed *(freely available)*
  www.indmed.nic.in/indmed.html
  This database covers peer-reviewed Indian biomedical journals.
- LILACS *(freely available)*
  www.lilacs.bvsalud.org/en/
  This database is a comprehensive index of scientific and technical literature about Latin America and the Caribbean.
- Medline *(subscription required)*/PubMed *(freely available)*
  www.pubmed.gov
  Medline and PubMed have the same content, made up of more than 22 million citations from biomedical literature, journals and online books.
- PDQ-Evidence for Informed Health Policymaking *(freely available)*
  www.pdq-evidence.org/
  PDQ ('pretty darn quick') Evidence includes systematic reviews, overviews of reviews, evidence-based policy briefs, primary studies and structured summaries of evidence for decisions about health systems.
- PEDro *(freely available)*
  www.pedro.org.au/
  PEDro contains over 23 000 randomised trials, systematic reviews and clinical practice guidelines in physiotherapy.
- PsycINFO *(subscription required)*
  This resource contains abstracts of articles and book chapters on behavioural sciences and mental health, and psychological aspects of related disciplines, such as management and learning.
- Social Care Online *(freely available)*
  www.scie-socialcareonline.org.uk/

Nowadays, with health and social care integrated, it is important to include social care evidence where appropriate. This database is the UK's largest database of information and research on all aspects of social care and social work.

Chapter 8: Searching healthcare databases

Grey literature

This is research that is not hosted in the usual ways, for example clinical databases, so it can be difficult to find. However, if you are carrying out a systematic review, then it is important that you identify grey literature as part of that research. Examples of grey literature include conference papers, theses, reports, bibliographies, unpublished work, research reports, and doctoral dissertations etc. Conference papers are now being indexed in Embase, and OpenGrey www.opengrey.eu/ is the System for Information on Grey Literature in Europe. It provides open access to 700 000 bibliographical references of grey literature produced in Europe.

Professional organisations

Institutions such as the Royal College of Nursing, Royal College of Surgeons, Chartered Society of Physiotherapy, etc. can often be found to be in the process of creating guidelines which have not yet been publicised on central guidelines databases. Yahoo has created a directory of professional organisations around the world:
www.dir.yahoo.com/Health/Medicine/Organizations/Professional/

Networks and colleagues

There are many clinical networks where people working with a similar goal can share ideas and learn from each other, and likewise, there are the local networks in which you practice. You must be aware of the potential biases with asking colleagues, as they might not be expert in the field, or the knowledge they have may be too localised or out of date. Formal networks are available:

- **The Cochrane Collaboration**
  The Cochrane Collaboration has groups and centres around the world. Each group has a web page so that you can see what work is in progress.
    www.cochrane.org/contact

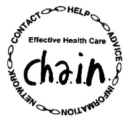

- **CHAIN (Contact, Help, Advice and Information Networks)**
  These are online networks for people working in health and social care. They are cross discipline and based around specific areas of interest, such as quality improvement, better care without delays, and patient and public involvement. These networks give people a simple and informal way of contacting each other to exchange ideas and share knowledge.

CHAIN England
   www.chain.ulcc.ac.uk/chain/index.html
CHAIN Canada
   www.epoc.uottawa.ca/CHAINCanada/

- **NHS Networks**
  This was developed to facilitate networking in the health service, enabling NHS staff across disciplines to share ideas and experiences and to improve the health service for those who work in it and use it.
   www.networks.nhs.uk

CHAPTER 4
Searching the Internet

When all else fails, you may need to search the Internet, a huge collection of knowledge and information on all topics, created by a range of authors, both expert and non-expert. It is difficult to tell which resources are more reliable than others, particularly when searching for health-related information. This chapter will provide guidance to facilitate effective Internet searching.

Advantages	Disadvantages
The World Wide Web is available 24 hours a day, 7 days a week	There is no guarantee of quality, accuracy or reliability as anybody can write for the World Wide Web, be they expert or amateur
Information can be very up to date	Unless the site is maintained on a regular basis, the information can quickly go out of date
Access is available to full text and unpublished information	Different search methods can make it difficult to find the information required

Search engines and directories
Search engines allow you to search through the 25 billion web pages to find information matching your criteria. Search engines are managed by robots, while directories are managed by human editors. No one engine searches the entire Internet, and therefore if you are carrying out a comprehensive search using the Internet, you should search using at least four search engines.

Google www.google.co.uk and MSN www.uk.msn.com/ are examples of search engines, while Yahoo www.uk.yahoo.com/ is a good example of a directory. The benefit of using a directory is that the content has been organised, so it can be easier to browse.

Basic searching
All search engines require the input of appropriate keywords or phrases. For example, if you want to find some information on clinical trials in diabetes for children, your keywords would be: diabetes children clinical trials. Typing

Searching Skills Toolkit: Finding the Evidence, Second Edition. Caroline De Brún and Nicola Pearce-Smith.
© 2014 John Wiley & Sons, Ltd. Published 2014 by John Wiley & Sons, Ltd.

these keywords into Google www.google.co.uk quickly retrieves web pages containing all the these words – note that the search retrieves over 14 million results.

You can use phrase searching to reduce the number of pages retrieved, for example typing: diabetes children 'clinical trials' will only retrieve pages with the exact phrase 'clinical trials', as well as the words diabetes and children.

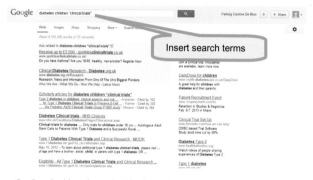

On Google this reduces the hits, but still retrieves around 9 million results, not to mention the adverts. Using a search engine will invariably retrieve tens of thousands of results, so try to use as many keywords as possible, or try using the Advanced Search facility.

The quality of the material found on the Web varies enormously, so you should consider any information carefully before using it. There are techniques and tools to help with appraising online health information and these are described further on.

Using a general search engine for finding health information is not usually recommended as a first port of call unless the condition is very rare, or you want to do some background research to get ideas for a more focused search.

Advanced searching

Many search engines have an advanced search facility, which allow the application of limits to the search, enabling you to narrow by type of publication (randomised controlled trial), date of publication, country, language, organisation type etc., just like a clinical database. This enables you to refine your search, thus avoiding overwhelming results.

With Advanced Search, you can limit your search to pages:

• that contain ALL the search terms you type in
• that contain the exact word or phrase you type in

- that contain at least one of the words you type in
- that do NOT contain any of the words you type in
- created in a certain file format
- that have been updated within a certain period of time
- within a certain domain, or website.

Yahoo Advanced Search
www.uk.search.yahoo.com/web/advanced

Google offers a research version of its search engine, called Google Scholar (www.scholar.google.co.uk/), which provides a simple way to search for research papers, articles, theses, books, opinions from professional societies, and online repositories. While easy to use, it should be used with caution when researching clinical queries, as it may not be completely up to date.

Tutorials

With websites that are specifically designed to search for information, there are often very good tutorials available. Check in the Help sections of individual search engines and online databases for more guidance on how to search effectively.

Evaluating material found on the World Wide Web

Researchers should be aware of some of the pitfalls involved with searching the Internet. Silberg et al. (1997)[8] published some guidance on appraising material found on the Internet. Simple questions should be considered, such as:

1. **Authorship** – Who wrote the research? Are they qualified? Where has the funding come from? Is there any bias?
2. **Attribution** – Is there any copyright information on the website? What is the source of the information?
3. **Disclosure** – Is it clear who owns the website? Could it be an organisation with a conflict of interest, e.g. medical supplier?
4. **Currency** – Is it clear when the research was written? Is it still relevant?
5. **Content** – Is it relevant to the population being researched? Is it accurate?

Anyone with a computer and access to some 'web space' can create a website to put up information on any topic. This information will be of variable quality because the Internet has no quality-control mechanisms. Therefore, information found on the Internet, especially about health and medical issues, should never be taken at face value. Some assessment of the validity and reliability of the information should be undertaken.

There are various evaluated, published criteria that can be used to help you assess the quality of health information found on websites, some of which are listed:

- *DISCERN instrument* – 16 questions to assess the quality of written information on treatment choices for a health problem.
  www.discern.org.uk/
- *Health on the Net Code of Conduct (HONcode)* – eight principles for assessing the quality and trustworthiness of health information on the Internet.
  www.hon.ch/HONcode/Pro/Visitor/visitor.html
- *International Patient Decision Aids Standards Instrument (IPDASi)* – a checklist of criteria to assess the quality of patient decision aids.
  www.ipdasi.org/2006%20IPDAS%20Quality%20Checklist.pdf

---

[8]Silberg, W.M., Lundberg, G.D. & Musacchio, R.A. 1997. Assessing, controlling, and assuring the quality of medical information on the Internet: Caveant lector et viewor—Let the reader and viewer beware. *JAMA*, 277(15), 1244–1245.

These, or similar criteria should be used to assess any medical or health information found from unappraised website sources, such as those sites retrieved in a general search of the Internet using Bing, Google or Yahoo.

Other good quality Internet sources of information

There is so much information on the Internet that it is vital to have a list of trusted websites to hand (the easiest way is to keep a list of 'Favourites' on Internet browser or on a social bookmarking resource – see the end of this chapter). The following is a list of additional Internet sites for a range of disciplines and languages:

Cross-discipline
- Ask Medline
  www.askmedline.nlm.nih.gov/ask/ask.php
- Best Bets
  www.bestbets.org/index.php
- BMJ specialty collections
  www.bmj.com/specialties
- *Clinical Evidence*
  www.clinicalevidence.bmj.com/x/index.html
- Campbell Collaboration
  www.campbellcollaboration.org/
- ClinicalTrials.gov
  www.clinicaltrials.gov/
- Current Controlled Trials
  www.controlled-trials.com/
- HONsearch – from Health On the Net Foundation (HON)
  www.hon.ch/HONsearch/Patients/medhunt.html
- PubMed PICO search
  www.pubmedhh.nlm.nih.gov/nlmd/pico/piconew.php

Search MEDLINE/PubMed via PICO with Spelling Checker
Patient, Intervention, Comparison, Outcome
go.usa.gov/xFn

Patient/Problem:

Medical condition:

> common cold

Intervention:
(therapy, diagnostic test, etc.)

> vitamin c

Compare to:
(same as above, optional):

> echinachea

Outcome:
(optional)

> improvement

Select Publication type:

> Not specified ▾

> Submit   Clear

- SUMSearch 2
  www.sumsearch.org/
- TRIP Database
  www.tripdatabase.com/

Midwifery and Nursing
- Evidence based nursing practice
  www.ebnp.co.uk/What%20is%20EBP.htm
- Intute – Midwifery
  www.vtstutorials.co.uk/tutorial/midwifery
- Intute – Nursing
  www.vtstutorials.co.uk/tutorial/nursing
- Introduction to evidence-based nursing
  www.cebm.utoronto.ca/syllabi/nur/intro.htm
- *Journal of Evidence-Based Nursing*
  www.ebn.bmj.com/

Public Health
- Centers for Disease Control and Prevention's (CDC's) WONDER (Wide-ranging Online Data for Epidemiologic Research) – database
  www.wonder.cdc.gov/

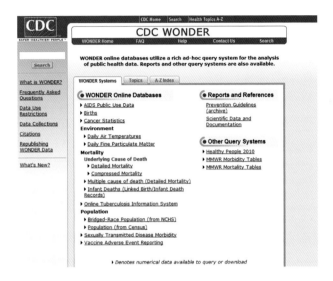

- Centers for Disease Control and Prevention
  www.cdc.gov
- E-roadmap to evidence-based public health practice
  www.health.ny.gov/prevention/prevention_agenda/evidence_based_
  public_health.htm
- Evidence-based practice for public health
  www.library.umassmed.edu/ebpph/index.cfm
- WHO Global Health Atlas
  www.who.int/GlobalAtlas
- World Health Organization
  www.who.int

Patient information
- CAPHIS (Consumer and Patient Health Information Section)
  www.caphis.mlanet.org/consumer/
- Department of Health Information Standard
  www.theinformationstandard.org/
- EQUIP – foreign language patient information
  www.equip.nhs.uk/language.html
- Health On the Net Foundation
  www.hon.ch/

- Henry Ford Health System Health Encyclopedia
  www.henryford.com/body.cfm?id=39115
- Health Finder
  www.healthfinder.gov/HealthTopics/
- NHS Choices
  www.nhs.uk/Conditions/Pages/hub.aspx
- Patient.co.uk
  www.patient.co.uk/

Glossaries
- EBM terms
  www.cebm.utoronto.ca/glossary/index.htm#top
- Evidence-based practice
  www.hsl.lib.umn.edu/learn/ebp/

Formulating clinical questions
- PubMed PICO
  www.pubmedhh.nlm.nih.gov/nlmd/pico/piconew.php
- Well-built clinical question
  www.hsl.lib.umn.edu/biomed/help/well-built-clinical-question

Non-English language sites
Healthcare is international, and there are many quality health resources available in different languages:
- **Chinese:**
  - Cochrane Collaboration
    www.ebm.org.cn
- **French:**
  - Canadian Health Service Research Foundation
    www.fcrss.ca/Home.aspx
  - Catalogue et Index des Sites Médicaux Francophones (CISMeF)
    www.cismef.org/
  - Cochrane Collaboration
    www.fr.cochrane.org/
  - Critique et pratique
    www.cetp.fmed.ulaval.ca/cetp/
- **German:**
  - Cochrane Collaboration
    www.cochrane.de/de/willkommen-auf-unseren-webseiten
  - Deutsches Netzwerk Evidenzbasierte Medizin e.V.
    www.ebm-netzwerk.de/
  - Horten-Zentrum für praxisorientierte Forschung und Wissenstransfer
    www.evimed.ch/

- **Iran:**
  ○ Iranian Centre for Evidence Based Medicine
    www.ircebm.tbzmed.ac.ir/
- **Italian:**
  ○ Gruppo Italiano per la Medicina Basata sulle Evidenze
    www.gimbe.org/
- **Spanish:**
  ○ Atrapando la evidencia
    www.infodoctor.org/rafabravo/netting.htm
  ○ Bandolera – Bandolier in Spanish
    www.infodoctor.org/bandolera/
  ○ EBP resources – Spanish
    www.fisterra.com/
  ○ Cochrane Collaboration
    www.update-software.com/clibplus/clibplus.asp
  ○ Instituto Argentino de Medicina Basada en las Evidencias
    www.iambe.org.ar/
  ○ CASPe
    www.redcaspe.org/drupal/

Programa de habilidades
en lectura crítica
España

Inicio | Contactos | Enlaces | Herramientas | Próximos Talleres | Mapa de la web | Buscador

Centres for Evidence-Based Practice:
- Critical Appraisal Skills Programme (CASP) Oxford
  www.casp-uk.net/
- Centre for Evidence Based Dentistry
  www.cebd.org/
- Centre for Evidence Based Dermatology
  www.nottingham.ac.uk/scs/divisions/evidencebaseddermatology/
  index.aspx
- Centre for Evidence Based Medicine – England
  www.cebm.net/
- Centre for Evidence-Based Medicine – Canada
  www.ktclearinghouse.ca/cebm/
- Centre for Evidence Based Mental Health
  www.cebmh.com/
- Evidence for Policy and Practice Information and Co-ordinating Centre
  www.eppi.ioe.ac.uk/cms/

Current Awareness Services:
- E-Watch Newsletter on Health Innovation
  www.santepop.qc.ca/en/activites/eveille.html

- Minervation National Elf Service
  www.nationalelfservice.net/
- QIPP @lert
  www.qippalert.blogspot.co.uk/

Saving useful websites

When searching the World Wide Web, it is worth building a collection of the best quality resources, so that they are always on hand when needed. There are two ways to do this:

Favourites and bookmarks

Your Internet browser, be it Internet Explorer, Firefox, Safari or Chrome, will have a facility allowing you to save important web addresses or Uniform Resource Locators (URLs). This means that you don't have to keep on typing in the address when you want to access that page.

Internet Explorer calls this facility 'Add to favourites'. In **Safari**, you can add bookmarks by clicking on the little cross to the left of the URL address book.

Firefox has the option to go to the Bookmarks menu and click on 'Bookmark this page'.

On **Google Chrome**, there is the option to click on the star to the right of the URL address book, where you can choose which bookmark folder to put it into. Once the bookmark is added, the star turns yellow.

Within these facilities, you can organise your favourites into folders, naming them to suit your requirements. There is also the option to have your key resources visible on a toolbar on your browser.

One problem with this storage facility is if you use different computers in different locations. These favourites or bookmarks stay on the computer where they have been set up although some browsers do let you create profiles so that you can access your bookmarks on other computers.

Online storage tools

Online tools have been developed so that you can access your favourite web resources on whichever computer you are using. This is known as Social Bookmarking as it allows bookmarks to be shared with colleagues and other like-minded people. One example is **Diigo** www.diigo.com/. This website allows people to save the Internet resources they use the most, tag them and share them with colleagues, or access them from whichever computer they are using. It means that you can save all your favourite websites, and access them wherever you are working.

Things to remember when searching the Internet:
- There are no controls over quality, although there are websites that have been developed with quality standards
- Users rarely go past the first page of hits on search engines such as Google
- Advertisers buy prominence on websites, in news media and in search engines
- Information may be biased, depending on who has published it
- Authorship and currency may be hard to determine
- Reliability is not the same as popularity nor indeed notoriety
- Individual search engines are not fully inclusive, so it is important to search more than one, and up to four, for comprehensive searches.

CHAPTER 5
Formulating searchable questions

Types of question

Clinical questions may be divided into background or foreground questions. A background question asks for general knowledge about a topic, and usually involves *who, what, when, why, where* or *how*.

> **Examples of background questions:**
> *What are the side effects of taking Drug A?*
> *What causes disease B?*
> *How is virus C transmitted?*

These sorts of questions can usually be answered by using textbooks, encyclopaedias, dictionaries or other reference sources.

A foreground question applies to specific patients or problems.

> **Examples of foreground questions:**
> *Will the use of acupuncture help a smoker of 30 years to quit smoking?*
> *Among children with hyperactivity disorder, does treatment with Ritalin affect symptoms?*
> *What is the risk of type II diabetes for adults who are obese and take little exercise?*

Foreground questions usually need to be answered by searching primary and secondary research literature, for example journal articles and other literature indexed in medical databases and online sources.

There are four main types of foreground question that are usually asked in healthcare:

Diagnosis – how those with and without a disease or condition can be distinguished

Harm – the side effects or disadvantages to an intervention

Prognosis – how the course of the disease or condition may progress

Treatment – effectiveness of interventions such as drugs, therapies, training or provision of information

Searching Skills Toolkit: Finding the Evidence, Second Edition. Caroline De Brún and Nicola Pearce-Smith.
© 2014 John Wiley & Sons, Ltd. Published 2014 by John Wiley & Sons, Ltd.

Why does this help you to search for evidence?
Knowing the type of question helps you to decide on the best type of research study to answer that question.

There are specific search terms or search filters (such as PubMed Clinical Queries) you can use for retrieving appropriate studies for each type of question – for more details see Chapter 9: Refining search results.

Breaking down the clinical scenario

The answer to a clinical question – the patient story – can be complicated to search for. By entering the entire scenario, it is unlikely that appropriate evidence will be found. The purpose of this section is to demonstrate methods for breaking down clinical scenarios to help health professionals find the best evidence available.

A clinical scenario arises from a meeting with a patient or perhaps from a gap in the research, but it is a question that is unanswered and needs to be resolved. The concept of breaking down the scenario, involves identifying the keywords. This enables you to turn a complicated case description into a more manageable question, making it easier to construct an effective search strategy.

PICO[9] is a popular method of managing a clinical question. The acronym stands for:

P	Patient/Problem/Population – meaning the individual, the condition or the group that is the subject of the clinical question
I	Intervention – the treatment that might be applied to the patient, problem, or population
C	Comparison – an alternative treatment that might provide similar if not greater benefits to the intervention. Please note: there may not always be a comparative intervention
O	Outcome – the expected result of the intervention (sometimes referred to as Exposure)

Here is an example of a clinical scenario:

> *A girl in her early twenties is being treated at your surgery for Myalgic Encephalomyelitis (ME). Her symptoms are extreme tiredness, pain, mood swings and night sweats. She has been prescribed Prozac, but would like to know if there are any alternative therapies that might relieve some or all of the symptoms associated with ME.*

[9]Sackett, D.L., Richardson, W.S., Rosenberg, W., Haynes, R.B. 1997. *Evidence-based medicine: how to practice and teach EBM*. Churchill Livingstone, New York.

Identifying keywords

The clinical scenario that has just been given is far too complicated to type into a search engine. So, the first stage of the clinical question formulation process is to identify the most important words – the keywords that will formulate the question. In this scenario, the keywords/phrases are underlined, shown as:

> A **girl in her early twenties** is being treated at your surgery for **Myalgic Encephalomyelitis (ME)**. Her symptoms are **extreme tiredness**, **pain**, **mood swings** and **night sweats**. She has been prescribed **Prozac**, but would like to know if there are any **alternative therapies** that might **relieve some or all of the symptoms** associated with ME.

So, from this scenario, we have:
- Age – 'girl in her early twenties' = young woman
- **P**roblem – Myalgic Encephalomyelitis
- **I**ntervention – Prozac
- **C**omparison – alternative medicine
- **O**utcome – relief of all or some of her symptoms.

Once the keywords/phrases are identified, a **simple**, **focused**, **clinical question** can be formulated, as follows:

> A **young woman** suffering from **Myalgic Encephalomyelitis**, has been prescribed **Prozac** but would like to know whether **alternative therapies** might provide **symptom relief**?

From this clinical question, the keywords can be put into a PICO table:

Patient/Problem	Intervention	Comparison	Outcome
Myalgic encephalomyelitis	Prozac	Alternative therapies	Symptom relief

Further reading

Huang, X., Lin, J. & Demner-Fushman, D. 2006. Evaluation of PICO as a knowledge representation for clinical questions. *AMIA Annu Symp Proc*, 359–363 available from: PM:17238363
✓**Full text:** www.ncbi.nlm.nih.gov/pmc/articles/PMC1839740/pdf/AMIA2006_0359.pdf

Richardson, W.S., Wilson, M.C., Nishikawa, J. & Hayward, R.S. 1995. The well-built clinical question: a key to evidence-based decisions. *ACP J Club*, 123(3), A12–A13 available from: PM:7582737
✓**Full text:**
www.eno.duhs.duke.edu/sites/eno.duhs.duke.edu/files/public/guides/richardson.pdf

Schardt, C., Adams, M.B., Owens, T., Keitz, S. & Fontelo, P. 2007. Utilization of the PICO framework to improve searching PubMed for clinical questions. *BMC Med Inform Decis Mak*, 7, 16 available from: PM:17573961
✓**Full text:** www.ncbi.nlm.nih.gov/pmc/articles/PMC1904193/

CHAPTER 6
Building a search strategy

Searching for evidence is a bit like going shopping. If you don't make a shopping list, you might forget to buy something you really need. When searching for evidence, if you don't make a list of all applicable terms, you might miss out on a key piece of research.

Identifying synonyms
The next stage is to compile a list of synonyms for each of the keywords. There are three things to think about:

Spelling	Research published in English may have spelling differences, depending on whether it is UK English or US English
Terminology	Different databases use different indexing terms. Medline and CINAHL index's use the term Allied Health Personnel, while Embase uses Paramedical Personnel for paramedics
Colloquial phrases	Deep vein thrombosis is sometimes referred to as 'economy-class syndrome', while bird flu is also known as avian influenza, or fowl plague

For a comprehensive search of the evidence, it is essential that all the alternative terms, spellings and acronyms are added to the PICO framework. Using the previous scenario of the young woman with ME, see example:

P	I	C	O
Myalgic encephalomyelitis	Antidepressants	Alternative therapy/medicine	Symptom relief
ME	Fluoxetine	Complementary therapy/medicine	Pain relief
Post viral fatigue syndrome	Prozac	Homoeopathy	Balanced moods
Chronic fatigue syndrome		Reflexology	Calm sleep
Yuppie flu		Nutritional/diet therapy	Increase in energy levels

Searching Skills Toolkit: Finding the Evidence, Second Edition. Caroline De Brún and Nicola Pearce-Smith.
© 2014 John Wiley & Sons, Ltd. Published 2014 by John Wiley & Sons, Ltd.

Synonym sources

When looking for synonyms, you might find it useful to do some background research into the condition. Sources might include:

- medical encyclopedias / dictionaries – looking up definitions may reveal alternative terms for the condition or symptoms
- colleagues – discussing the condition with colleagues, particularly those from overseas, may bring up terms which you had not thought of or perhaps even come across before
- patient information – reliable patient information sources may be able to provide you with useful terms that you might want to build into your search strategy.

Truncation and wildcards

Truncation and wildcards are handy little shortcuts for **free-text** searching, which can substantially reduce the number of search terms that need to be added.

Truncation

Truncation allows the use of a symbol, usually an asterisk * or a dollar sign $ to expand the search, by taking the stem of a word and adding the symbol at the end – so, child* or child$ will search for child, children, childhood etc.

If your search involves the keyword 'ulcers' or 'ulceration', you could type in ulcer, ulcers, ulceration, ulcerated, ulcerative etc., or you could save time by typing in either:

- ulcer* – which searches for ulcer, ulcers, ulceration, ulcerated, ulcerative in PubMed
- ulcer$ – which searches for ulcer, ulcers, ulceration, ulcerated, ulcerative in Ovid Medline and Dialog Medline
- ulcer$2 – which takes the stem of the word, e.g. ulcer and searches for one or two-letter endings, therefore, ulcer or ulcers but not ulceration, ulcerated or ulcerative.

This reduces the number of search steps, while increasing the number of hits. However, when using truncation, it is important to remember the differences in spelling. For example, the word 'stabilising', could also be spelt 'stabilizing', so if one uses truncation, one would need to ensure that either both terms are searched for using truncation or a shorter stem is used, e.g. stabili$ – this would look for stabilising, stabilizing and stability.

CAUTION!
Do not use too short a stem as the search will become too broad, and not retrieve relevant records. For example: car* or car$ will find care, careful, cardiology, carcinogenic etc.

Wildcards
British English and American English sometimes
have different spellings, for example:

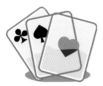

British English	American English
paediatric	pediatric
behaviour	behavior
colour	color

Wildcards usually come in the form of a question mark. So, instead of typing in both terms, a question mark is inserted in place of the extra letter, e.g. p?ediatric, behavio?r, colo?r, and this will search for the occurrence of the British English spelling or the American English spelling.

Wildcards are also useful for dealing with plurals, such as woman or women. You can just type wom?n to retrieve both.

If you aren't sure whether a hyphen is present, then use a wildcard. For example, intra?operative will retrieve papers on intraoperative and intra-operative.

Use the Help Pages for individual databases to find out whether they apply truncation and/or wildcards, and if yes, which ones they use and how.

Table 6.1 summarises which forms of truncation, wildcards, and Boolean operators are used by each database provider.

Table 6.1 Summary or truncation, wildcards, and Boolean operators
Remember: each software provider has a Help facility to provide further guidance on searching.

Symbol	Definition	Cochrane	Dialog	EBSCO	Ovid	ProQuest	PubMed
*	All words beginning with a particular stem e.g. nurs*	✓	✓	✓		✓	✓
$	All words beginning with a particular stem e.g. nurs$		✓	✓	✓		
:	All words beginning with a particular stem e.g. nurs:			✓	✓	✓	
?	Replaces exactly the number of characters specified by the number of ? used e.g. nurs?, nurs???		✓				
*	All words ending with the same root e.g. *glycemic (hypo or hyper)	✓					
*	Overcoming spelling differences and searching for singular and plural e.g. colo*r	✓	✓				
#	Overcoming spelling differences and searching for singular and plural e.g. colo#r			✓	✓		
?	Overcoming spelling differences and searching for singular and plurals e.g. colo?r.		✓	✓	✓		
*	Use between words to match any word			✓			
AND	For all the words	✓	✓	✓	✓		✓
OR	Searches for at least one of the words in the search string	✓	✓	✓	✓		✓

Symbol	Definition	Cochrane	Dialog	EBSCO	Ovid	ProQuest	PubMed
NOT	Excludes a word from the search	✓	✓	✓	✓		✓
-	For words next together, in the order specified.	✓					✓
""	Phrase searching – groups words together in the order specified	✓		✓	✓		✓
( )	Phrase searching – groups words together in the order specified		✓	✓	✓		
ADJ	For words next together or within x words of each other, in the order specified				✓		
NEXT	For the 1st word with the 2nd following within the next x words	✓					
NEAR	For the 1st word and the 2nd in either order, within the next x words	✓				✓	
N	For the 1st word and the 2nd in either order, within the next x words			✓			
W	Within x number of words and in the order entered			✓			
FREQ	Searches for a specified number of times the word appears in the record				✓		

Combining terms (using Boolean operators)

The process of building a search strategy involves the use of 'Boolean operators'. These are words which combine the terms that have been selected for the search, making the search more relevant to the clinical question. Table 6.2 shows the Boolean operators available and the definition of each:

Table 6.2 Definitions of Boolean operators

Boolean operator	Definition
and/AND	Narrows the search results; all terms are searched for e.g. measles AND children AND adults
or/OR	Broadens the search results, one or more of the search terms are found, e.g. venous thrombosis OR DVT OR deep vein thrombosis
not/NOT	Limits the searches by restricting the terminology searched for, e.g. children NOT adults. Use this with caution, as it would exclude papers about children <u>and</u> adults
adj/ADJ	Searches for all the words side by side (adjacent), as a phrase, in any order, e.g. deep ADJ1 vein ADJ1 thrombosis. If you add a number after 'ADJ', the database searches for all occurrences where the two words appear separated by the number of words matching the number, e.g. chronic ADJ3 syndrome, would find 'chronic fatigue syndrome' and 'chronic fatigue immune deficiency syndrome'
()	Brackets can be used in two ways: **1)** when combining with two Boolean operators, e.g. measles AND (children OR adults), so the database will look for articles about children or adults with measles **2)** when searching for a phrase – some databases use brackets, e.g. (assertive community treatment)
""	By putting the keywords in inverted commas, some databases will search for the words as phrases, e.g. "assertive community treatment"

Venn diagrams of common Boolean operators:

AND

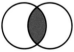 Searching for diabetes AND insulin will retrieve only those resources containing both words (the pink-shaded section).

OR

Searching for antidepressants OR counselling will retrieve resources containing either term, or both (the pink-shaded section).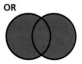

NOT

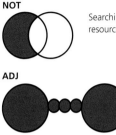

Searching for contraception NOT oral would exclude resources containing the word oral.

ADJ

This is used to search for words in a specific order, as a phrase, e.g. deep ADJ3 thrombosis will retrieve deep vein thrombosis and deep venous thrombosis.

Some databases will insist that the Boolean operators are upper case, whereas with other databases it does not matter whether they are upper or lower case. All databases and search engines will have tips or help pages, so you can check out their policy on case sensitivity. The key point is to remember how they are used so that you can apply them effectively.

Boolean operators connect your search terms together, enabling you to find the most relevant references to answer your clinical questions. Some databases do use other Boolean operators, but the ones mentioned previously are the key ones.

Table 6.1 specifies which databases use which Boolean operators, wildcards and truncation.

If you do not get the results you are looking for, double check your search strategy to see whether there are any spelling mistakes or errors in Boolean operator application (e.g. did you use OR instead of AND?).

Seek advice: your local medical librarian is a fresh pair of eyes who can review your search strategy.

Construction of the final search strategy

Using the PICO table developed at the beginning of this chapter, along with our knowledge of Boolean operators we can now construct our search strategy in two stages.

Stage one involves combining the terms under each heading, (P, I, C and then O) with **OR**. It is not necessary to find articles containing all of these words, just articles that contain one or more of the terms.

For example:

STAGE ONE			
P	I	C	O
Myalgic encephalomyelitis **OR** ME **OR** Post viral fatigue syndrome **OR** Chronic fatigue syndrome **OR** Yuppie flu	Antidepressants **OR** Fluoxetine **OR** Prozac	Alternative therapy/medicine **OR** Complementary therapy/medicine **OR** Homoeopathy **OR** Reflexology **OR** Nutritional/diet therapy	Symptom relief **OR** Pain relief **OR** Balanced moods **OR** Calm sleep **OR** Increase in energy levels

So, the search process would involve searching for all the terms under column **P** first, combining each of them with OR, and then doing the same process for columns **I**, **C** (if appropriate) and **O**.

Once all the terms have been combined in their groups with OR you can go onto **Stage two**, which involves combining the groups (P,I,C and O) using AND. If there is no comparison intervention, there will be no need to add column C into the search strategy.

STAGE TWO						
P		I		C		O
Myalgic encephalomyelitis		Antidepressants		Alternative therapy/medicine		Symptom relief
	AND		**AND**		**AND**	

In summary, to develop an effective search strategy, one must:
1. breakdown the clinical scenario and formulate a more manageable question
2. identify the keywords and make a note of relevant synonyms
3. combine using appropriate Boolean concepts.

Sometimes you have to use brackets to distinguish between ANDs and ORs.

P	I
(Myalgic encephalomyelitis **OR** ME **OR** Post viral fatigue syndrome **OR** Yuppie flu**)** **AND** **(**Antidepressants **OR** Fluoxetine **OR** Prozac**)**	

Refining search strategies (also known as limiting)

In Chapter 8: Searching healthcare databases, there will be comprehensive descriptions for applying these search strategies to specific healthcare databases using different methods, such as free text and thesaurus.

Chapter 8: Searching healthcare databases ➤

Once the search has been carried out, if too many results have been retrieved, the search can be further restricted with the application of limits. Limits allow the search to be restricted in a number of ways, such as publication type, age and language – for more details see Chapter 9: Refining search results.

Chapter 9: Refining search results ➤

CHAPTER 7

Free text and thesaurus searching

You have now completed the first three steps of the search process:

1. **Decided on the question type and information source**
2. **Formulated a searchable question**
3. **Identified appropriate keywords and synonyms**

You are now ready to search for your evidence. You can do this using:
1. free text searching and
2. thesaurus searching.

Free text searching

Free text searching, also known as natural language searching, means that the database will search for exactly what you type into the box, in any field of a record. This is the natural way to search but not necessarily the most effective. There are pros and cons to the use of free text:

Pros	For example
Useful for unambiguous topics or new interventions not indexed elsewhere yet	If you type in 'assertive community treatment', the database will find papers specifically on this intervention
Brand names of drugs or proper names	If you type in Prozac, the database will find papers about Prozac

Cons	For example
Too many irrelevant results	If you type in diabetes, the database will search for every occurrence of the word diabetes and retrieve an unmanageable amount of results, many of which will only have a minor reference to diabetes
Disregards plurals	If you are looking for research on disability and you type in disability, the database will look for disability but not disabilities, so you will miss out on important research
Ignores spelling differences	If you are searching for papers on behaviour (British English) you will miss out on research on behavior (American English)

Searching Skills Toolkit: Finding the Evidence, Second Edition. Caroline De Brún and Nicola Pearce-Smith.
© 2014 John Wiley & Sons, Ltd. Published 2014 by John Wiley & Sons, Ltd.

To lower the number of hits you can field search, for example search only in the title or the title and abstract. This will make the search more specific, but you may miss out on key papers because you are not aware of all the relevant synonyms. A more effective way of searching uses a thesaurus.

Thesaurus searching

To ensure that no literature is missed, it is important to recognise the existence of different spelling and variances in terminology for the same search topics. For example, deep vein thrombosis is known by many names, including DVT, economy-class syndrome and venous thrombosis. Articles may use any of these words to describe DVT, and it is not always possible to know all the synonyms.

One way to overcome these differences when searching a database is to use the thesaurus. A thesaurus can be referred to in many ways:
- MeSH, in the database Medline (see Advanced MeSH searching further on in this chapter, and Chapter 8: Searching healthcare databases)
- controlled vocabulary
- descriptor
- subject headings
- keyword
- index term.

A thesaurus is a collection of terms that have been developed for a particular database – each record contained in the database is assigned several of these thesaurus terms (usually between 5 and 20) in order to identify the key themes or subjects it covers. Shown here is an example of the MeSH terms that have been assigned to a Medline (PubMed) record.

MeSH Terms
Adult
Blood Glucose/analysis
Diabetes Mellitus, Type 1/diagnosis
Diabetes Mellitus, Type 1/drug therapy*
Diabetes Mellitus, Type 2/diagnosis
Diabetes Mellitus, Type 2/drug therapy*
Dose-Response Relationship, Drug
Drug Administration Schedule
Female
Fetal Development/drug effects
Gestational Age
Humans
Insulin/therapeutic use*
Insulin Infusion Systems
Pregnancy

This means that articles on the same topic should be assigned the same thesaurus terms, regardless of how the subject is described in the text of the article. Therefore, searching a database using specific thesaurus terms aids the retrieval of records on the same topic. The main difference with searching using thesaurus terms is that the articles you find will be *specifically* about the topic you are searching for – searching for a term using free text will find articles containing the word or words somewhere in the article, and will not necessarily be specifically about the topic you are interested in.

Another good reason for searching the thesaurus is that one term often incorporates a range of synonyms. For example, the MeSH 'Venous Thrombosis' also searches for papers specifically on venous thromboses, deep vein thrombosis, DVT, and phlebothrombosis or phlebothromboses, so it saves you having to type all those terms in.

Thesaurus searching also overcomes the problem of different spellings and different terminology. For example, searching using the MeSH 'Fetal Diseases' will also retrieve papers containing 'foetal diseases', and using MeSH 'Allied Health Personnel' should retrieve papers about physiotherapists, physician assistants, paramedics etc, provided that these articles have been correctly indexed.

Thesaurus searching is the most efficient way of searching as you can find articles of relevance, and you save time by keying in fewer terms, although you will need to think of all the MeSH terms for each concept. For example, with the MeSH term 'Pregnancy', you may also want to include the following index terms: 'Pregnant women', 'Pregnancy complications', and 'Prenatal care'. You should be aware that not all indexing is 100% accurate (due to human error), and not all entries in a database will be adequately indexed in sufficient detail.

Additionally, not all articles entered into a database will have index terms assigned immediately – for example, recent articles will be entered onto the PubMed database soon after publication, but there is usually a time gap before thesaurus terms are assigned. Restricting your search to a thesaurus search would therefore exclude recently published articles. A combination of thesaurus and free text searching with wildcards and truncation, will help to prevent relevant papers being missed.

Browsing and mapping

In most databases there are two ways to use the thesaurus – browsing or automatic mapping. In PubMed, you can:

1. browse the MeSH Database – this takes you to the thesaurus, and allows you to type in the term you are looking for, presenting you with a list of suitable terms. For example, typing 'deep vein thrombosis' into the MeSH Database will tell you that the term used in Medline is 'Venous Thrombosis'

2. use Mapping – when you type a term into the main search box, PubMed tries to automatically map your term to an appropriate MeSH – this will

then be included in your search. For example, typing 'deep vein thrombosis' into the search box will automatically map to the MeSH 'Venous Thrombosis' and include this in your search.

	CAUTION!
	PubMed will not be able to map all terms typed into the search box to a MeSH, so ideally you should check the MeSH database

Advanced MeSH searching

MeSH are organised into 'trees' so that you can see how the database is applying them. An example of a MeSH tree in PubMed is shown:

> All MeSH Categories
>> Diseases Category
>>> Cardiovascular Diseases
>>>> Vascular Diseases
>>>>> Embolism and Thrombosis
>>>>>> Thrombosis
>>>>>>> **Venous Thrombosis**
>>>>>>>> Budd-Chiari Syndrome
>>>>>>>> Postthrombotic Syndrome
>>>>>>>> Retinal Vein Occlusion
>>>>>>>> Thrombophlebitis
>>>>>>>>> Lemierre Syndrome
>>>>>>>> Upper Extremity Deep Vein Thrombosis

Explode and Single Term

The MeSH selected is in bold. Beneath the selected MeSH, there is an indented list of narrower terms. There is an option to 'Explode' the MeSH. This means that when the database searches for the MeSH, it will also search for the narrower terms below the MeSH, widening your options.

If you choose not to Explode the MeSH, the database will only search for the Single term (the MeSH that you have typed in). This can limit too much, and it is often best to keep the search broad and narrow it down by adding more search terms.

Focus

The Focus option is not available on all databases. It retrieves articles where your MeSH term is the primary focus of the article. This can be too restrictive, so use with caution.

Major and Minor Descriptors

Major Descriptors are the keywords that identify the main themes of the paper. Minor Descriptors are the keywords that identify the secondary themes of the paper.

Subheadings

Many databases allow you to narrow down your MeSH by choosing specific subheadings. While this is a useful option, it is often best to keep the search broad and narrow it down by adding the other concepts from your PICO framework.

Related terms

This is a useful feature because it allows you to see other MeSH which might also apply to your search. For example, the related term for 'fetal diseases' is 'congenital abnormalities', which you might not have thought to include in your search. The database does not automatically include Related terms in the search, but you can add it as an additional term to your search strategy.

CHAPTER 8
Searching healthcare databases

Finding the evidence: key steps

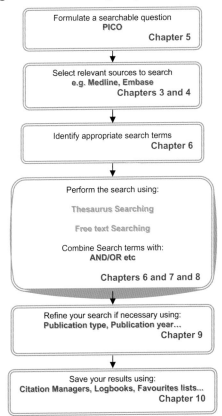

Searching Skills Toolkit: Finding the Evidence, Second Edition. Caroline De Brún and Nicola Pearce-Smith.
© 2014 John Wiley & Sons, Ltd. Published 2014 by John Wiley & Sons, Ltd.

Whichever resource you choose to search, the principles remain the same, as the flow chart shows. All searchable resources will have help sheets and/or tutorials available. Make use of these, and if you still need help, contact your local librarian. If unfamiliar with the information source, use the help pages/search tips of that resource – Chapter 8 and Appendix 1.

There are five main providers of healthcare databases:

1. Cochrane Collaboration – The Cochrane Library Database of Systematic Reviews, Database of Reviews of Effects, CENTRAL database of randomised controlled trials, Economic Evaluations Database, and Health Technology Assessments.
2. EBSCO – CINAHL, Medline, Health Business Elite, and Salud en Español.
3. National Library of Medicine – PubMed, free version of Medline.
4. Ovid Wolters Kluwer – Access to AMED, British Nursing Index, Embase, Medline and PsycINFO.
5. Proquest Dialog – Medline, Health Management, Hospital Collection, Nursing and Allied Health Source, PsycINFO, AMED, British Nursing Index, and Embase.

Greater detail about healthcare databases can be found in Chapter 3: Clinical information: sources. Further hints and tips on searching can be found in Chapter 7: Free text and thesaurus, and the present chapter.

This chapter will demonstrate the functionality of Ovid Medline, PubMed, CINAHL EBSCO, and the Cochrane Library to highlight the differences between interface designs, while demonstrating the similarities in use.

At the end of Chapter 6: Building a search strategy, there is a summary table detailing which forms for truncation, wildcards, and Boolean operators, each software provider uses.

To demonstrate how to perform a search on the two featured interfaces for Medline, we will use the same scenario. Note that we have included numbers of hits retrieved for example purposes, but these depend on the date of the search, how often the interface is updated and features such as automatic MeSH mapping – these will differ between interface and if the same search is repeated at a later date.

Scenario: A one-year-old child is admitted to the paediatrics department with bronchiolitis, where she is given a course of steroids. This prompts the doctor on duty to find out whether there is any evidence that corticosteroids lead to less hospital stays or improved recovery where bronchiolitis is concerned.

Focused question: Among young children with bronchiolitis, does treatment with corticosteroids lead to less hospital stays or improved recovery?

Problem	Intervention	Comparison	Outcome
bronchiolitis	corticosteroids **OR** steroids	none	stays **OR** hospitalisation **OR** improvement **OR** recovery

Type of question: Intervention/treatment
Best feasible study design: Systematic review or randomised controlled trial
Databases to search: Medline, Embase, CINAHL, Cochrane Library

Medline

Medline is the major bibliographic database for biomedical literature, and covers subjects such as medicine, dentistry, nursing and allied health. The database contains citations and abstracts from biomedical journals published in the USA, UK and many other countries.

Medline is provided electronically by a variety of publishers, three of which we cover in this chapter:
- PubMed (freely available)
- Ovid (subscription)
- EBSCO (subscription).

PubMed (www.pubmed.gov)

PubMed is provided by the National Library of Medicine (USA) and includes all the citations from MEDLINE. It is freely available to anyone with an Internet connection.

Search process

Can I just type 'bronchiolitis AND steroids' into the main search box?
Yes, but this retrieves 642 hits – do you want to look at them all?

PubMed tries to automatically map words to appropriate Medical Subject Headings – if this is possible, both the free text and the MeSH will be included in the search. Look at the 'Search details' box on the right-hand side of the PubMed screen, or see the section on Ovid Medline.

Try searching for a systematic review in Clinical Queries. Click on the Clinical Queries link to start and enter search terms:

This search retrieved 21 hits, including this systematic review: ***Steroids and bronchodilators for acute bronchiolitis in the first two years of life: systematic review and meta-analysis.*** Hartling L, Fernandes RM, Bialy L et al. BMJ. 2011 Apr 6;342:d1714.

> When using the filters on Clinical Queries, you are restricting your PubMed search quite considerably, so begin by using only the key terms, and by making your search quite broad (i.e. do not combine too many search terms together with 'AND'). If you make your search too narrow when using Clinical Queries you will retrieve very little. You can always narrow the search later.

If the Systematic reviews list does not yield satisfactory results, or you wish to expand the search, try restricting to 'Therapy' as type of question.

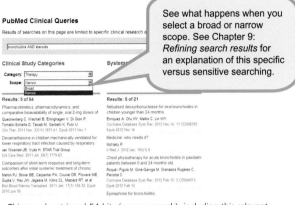

See what happens when you select a broad or narrow scope. See Chapter 9: *Refining search results* for an explanation of this specific versus sensitive searching.

This search retrieved 54 hits (narrow search), including this relevant randomised controlled trial: *Dexamethasone in children mechanically ventilated for lower respiratory tract infection caused by respiratory syncytial virus: a randomized controlled trial. van Woensel JB, Vyas H; STAR Trial Group. Crit Care Med. 2011 Jul;39(7):1779–83.*

What if using Clinical Queries has not retrieved any results that help me to answer my question?

You can broaden your search using the search techniques we learned in Chapter 7: Free text and thesaurus searching.

Chapter 7: Free text and thesaurus searching

Include a free text term and a MeSH for each relevant PICO term whenever possible.

Free text searching

Think of all the alternate spellings for free text, and make use of truncation (* symbol on PubMed) to expand word endings. For example:

hospitalisation OR hospitalization	Includes UK and US spellings
corticosteroid*	Finds corticosteroid (singular) and corticosteroids (plural)
improv*	Finds improve, improves, improved, improving etc.

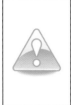 Be careful not to truncate too near the beginning of words, as you will retrieve too many different words. For example, *imp** will not only find the words, but also everything else beginning with *imp*. You will also find that if there are too many word endings, a message will appear stating *Wildcard search for imp** *used only the first 600 variations. Lengthen the root word to search for all endings*.

MeSH searching

The following example shows how to find the MeSH term for 'corticosteroids'.

1. Click on MeSH Database.
2. Type 'corticosteroids' into the search box.
3. Tick the box next to 'Adrenal Cortex Hormones'.
4. Click on 'Add to search builder', then 'Search PubMed' to perform the search.

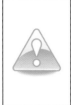

Relevant citations in Medline may be indexed with the MeSH 'Adrenal Cortex Hormones', or contain the free text word 'corticosteroids' in the title or abstract, (or all three).

It is important to include both MeSH and free text in your search, in case an article contains only one or the other.

Combining search terms

Free text and MeSH can be combined using Boolean logic (AND, OR).

Chapter 6: Building a search strategy

Combine similar concepts with OR to expand the search ('OR means more'). Combine different concepts with AND to narrow the search.

An example of a finished search strategy is shown here. Each line is numbered e.g. #1 – these line numbers can be used when combining searches. To see your search history, click on the 'Advanced' link under the PubMed search box. This search retrieved 391 hits.

> 3 different concepts combined with **AND** to give final result

> Similar concept (MeSH and free text) terms combined with **OR**

Viewing the results

Click on the number of hits next to the line you want to view, i.e. 391. The title and author details will be displayed in batches of 20 – to view more (or less) records on one page, click on the 'Display Settings' link, and choose the number of items per page. You can also sort the records by publication date, author or journal title using 'Display Settings'.

To see the abstract for an individual article, click on the Title. If you wish to see the abstracts of all articles in your search, click on the Display Settings menu and choose 'Abstract'.

If free full text is available, a link to 'Free article' or 'Free PMC [PubMed Central] article' is provided. PubMed Central www.ncbi.nlm.nih.gov/pmc/ is a free full text archive containing biomedical and life sciences journal articles.

Clipboard

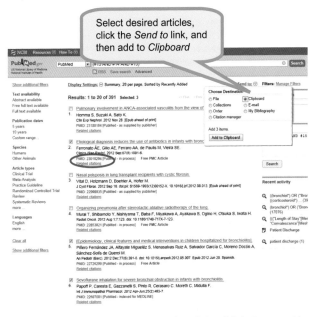

> Select desired articles, click the *Send to* link, and then add to *Clipboard*

To view the selected articles later, click on the 'Clipboard' link. You can add up to 500 records to the Clipboard – these will be lost after 8 hours of inactivity.

Related citations

Another way to find potentially relevant articles in PubMed is to use the 'Related citations' feature. When you find a relevant citation from your search, click on the 'Related citations' link under the citation, as shown. This will bring up a new list of articles that are 'related' (i.e. they have similar MeSH) to your chosen citation.

Saving or emailing records

Using the 'Send to' link you can choose what to do with your results, including generating a file for use in a citation manager, or choosing to *Email* them to yourself.

If you wish to import citations from PubMed into EndNote or Reference Manager, you will need to select 'Send to Citation Manager'. This allows you to save your citations in a format which can be imported into a Citation Manager (see Chapter 10: Saving citations).

Ovid Medline (www.ovid.com)

Ovid Technologies (part of Wolters Kluwer Health) provides an interface on the World Wide Web for searching the Medline database. It is a subscription service, often available via libraries, universities or hospitals.

Search process

Can I just type 'bronchiolitis AND steroids' into the Advanced search box? Yes, but this retrieves 227 hits – do you want to look at them all?

Try using Clinical Queries, and restricting to 'Reviews' or 'Therapy' as type of question. On the Advanced search page, type 'bronchiolitis AND steroids', then click the 'Search' button – after the search has been performed, click on 'Limits', then 'Additional Limits'.

Select the type of question, for example 'Reviews' or 'Therapy'.

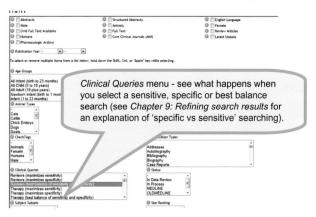

Clinical Queries menu - see what happens when you select a sensitive, specific or best balance search (see *Chapter 9: Refining search results* for an explanation of 'specific vs sensitive' searching).

The 'Reviews (best balance of sensitivity and specificity)' search retrieved 60 hits, including the systematic review by Hartling et al. These search filters are based on the ones by Haynes RB et al.[10] that are also used in PubMed Clinical Queries.

What if using Clinical Queries has not retrieved any results that help me to answer my question?

You can broaden your search using the search techniques we learned in Chapter 7.

Chapter 7: Free text and thesaurus searching

Include a free text term and a MeSH for each relevant PICO term whenever possible.

Free text
Think of all the alternate spellings for free text, and make use of truncation to expand word endings. The truncation symbol on Ovid is $ or *.

[10] *Summary of Enhancements for Clinical and Health Services Research Queries for PubMed for Studies.* 2011. Available from www.nlm.nih.gov/pubs/techbull/jf04/cq_info.html.

For example:

hospitalisation OR hospitali?ation	Includes UK and US spellings
corticosteroid$	Finds corticosteroid (singular) and corticosteroids (plural)
improv$	Finds improve, improves, improved, improving etc.

MeSH

PubMed tries to map all words automatically to appropriate MeSH – if this is possible, both the free text and the MeSH will be included in the search. PubMed will always default to 'Explode' the MeSH.

Ovid will also try to automatically map to appropriate MeSH, providing that the 'Map Term to Subject Heading' box is ticked. However, Ovid does not 'Explode' MeSH unless requested.

To make sure that you include both exploded MeSH and free text when using Ovid Medline, search each term separately – for example, type 'bronchiolitis' into the Advanced search box, make sure the 'Map Term to Subject Heading' box is selected, and click the Search button. Ovid will then display a list of possible MeSH, giving you the option to 'Explode', and to include the free text word:

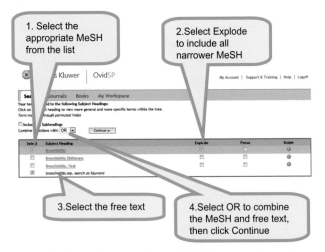

Repeat for the search term 'corticosteroids'. Finally, you need to combine the two different search concepts.

Combining search terms

Free text and MeSH can be combined using Boolean logic (AND, OR). More can be found on this concept in Chapter 6: Building a search strategy.

You can also type 1 AND 2 into the search box to combine the terms.

97 citations are retrieved – many of these are different from the ones you obtained when using Clinical Queries, as you are now searching the whole of Medline. This a way of broadening your search to retrieve more potentially relevant articles; however, you have to remember that lower quality study types will be also be retrieved, along with editorials and letters etc.

Viewing the results

Click on the 'Display' link next to the line you want to view. The title and author details will be displayed in batches of 100 – to view more (or less) records on one page, click on the '100 per page' menu and change the citations per page.

To see the abstract for an individual article, click 'View Abstract'. If there is a 'pdf' link next to the record, this means that electronic full text is available. Many of these full text articles will require a subscription (possibly available via your institution).

Printing, emailing or exporting records

You can choose to print, email or export your results. Select results by ticking the box next to the record.

> If you wish to export citations directly from Ovid Medline into a Citation Manager database (see Chapter 10: Saving citations), you will need to click on 'Export', and then select the desired resource, e.g. Reference Manager, Endnote, Procite, etc.

Find similar articles
Another way to find potentially relevant articles is to use the 'Find Similar' feature (like the 'Related citations' feature on PubMed).

Other databases available via Ovid
Ovid also provides access to other useful healthcare databases, such as:
- Embase – a biomedical and pharmacological database which is especially strong in its coverage of drug and pharmaceutical research
- PsycINFO (American Psychological Association database) – a database providing systematic coverage of the psychological literature from the 1800s to the present
- AMED (complementary medicines and alternative therapies database) – a database covering journals from professions allied to medicine, complementary medicine and palliative care
- HMIC (Health Management Information Consortium) – a database containing health and social care management/services information.

These databases have their own keyword indexes (similar to MeSH), and can be searched in the same way as above. There is some crossover of articles (especially between Medline and Embase), but all databases will also have many unique articles.

CINAHL (www.ebscohost.com/)
CINAHL is provided by EBSCOhost, and provides access to thousands of abstracts and hundreds of full text articles from nursing and allied health journals. Topics include nursing, biomedicine, health sciences, librarianship, alternative/complementary medicine, consumer health, and 17 allied health disciplines.

Problem	Intervention	Comparison	Outcome
Stroke **OR** cerebrovascular accident	rehabilitation **OR** physiotherapy **OR** physical therapy **OR** occupational therapy	none	quality of life **OR** improved speech **OR** improved movement

Scenario: A 55-year-old stroke sufferer wants to know whether rehabilitation will improve her quality of life.
Focused question: In stroke patients can rehabilitation improve quality of life?
Type of question: Intervention/treatment
Best feasible study design: Systematic review or randomised controlled trial
Databases to search: CINAHL, Medline, Cochrane Library

Search process
Can I just type 'stroke AND rehabilitation' into the main search box?
  Yes, but this retrieves 1511 hits – do you want to look at them all?

CINAHL will search just for 'stroke AND rehabilitation' and not include the other synonyms. There is the option to use Subject Terms to help find more relevant results which include the narrower terms, such as 'physical therapy' and 'occupational therapy' for rehabilitation.

You can improve your search using the search techniques we learned in Chapter 7: Free text and thesaurus searching.
Include a free text term and a Subject Term (MeSH version of CINAHL) for each relevant PICO term whenever possible.

Free text searching
Think of all the alternate spellings for free text, and make use of truncation (* symbol on CINAHL) to expand word endings. For example:

stroke*	Finds stroke (singular) and strokes (plural)
rehabilitat*	Finds rehab, rehabilitation, rehabilitate
improv*	Finds improve, improves, improved, improving etc.

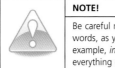

NOTE!
Be careful not to truncate too near the beginning of words, as you will retrieve too many different words. For example, *imp** will not only find the words, but also everything else beginning with *imp*.

Searching for Subject Terms

Subject Terms are the CINAHL version of MeSH. The following example shows how to find the Subject Term for 'rehabilitation':

1. Type in rehabilitation and tick the box 'Suggest Subject Terms', above the search box. Click on 'Search'.
2. Choose 'Rehabilitation' and tick the 'Explode' option to ensure that the narrower terms of 'occupational therapy', and 'physical therapy', are included.
3. Subheadings are automatically included.
4. Click on 'Search Database'.

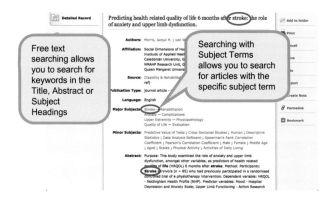

Relevant citations in CINAHL may be indexed with the Subject Term 'Stroke', or contain the free text word 'stroke' in the title or abstract, (or all three, as shown).

It is important to include both Subject Terms and free text in your search, in case an article contains only one or the other.

Combining search terms

Free text and Subject Terms can be combined using Boolean logic (AND, OR).

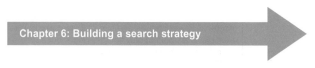

Chapter 6: Building a search strategy

Combine similar concepts with OR to expand the search ('OR means more'). Combine different concepts with AND to narrow the search.

An example of a finished search strategy is shown with the most recent search first, unlike other databases. This can easily be changed, by clicking on Search ID#, which changes the order of the searches. Each line is numbered, e.g. #1 – these line numbers can be used when combining searches.

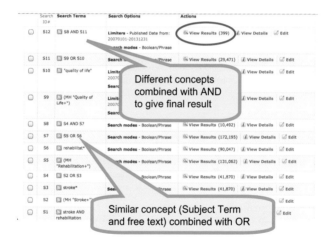

	Search ID#	Search Terms	Search Options	Actions		
○	S12	S8 AND S11	Limiters - Published Date from: 20070101-20131231 Search modes - Boolean/Phrase	View Results (399)	View Details	Edit
○	S11	S9 OR S10	Search ... /Phrase	View Results (29,471)	View Details	Edit
○	S10	"quality of life"	Limite... 2007... Search		View Details	Edit
○	S9	(MH "Quality of Life+")	Limit... 2007... Search		View Details	Edit
○	S8	S4 AND S7	Search modes - Boolean/Phrase	View Results (10,492)	View Details	Edit
○	S7	S5 OR S6	Search modes - Boolean/Phrase	View Results (172,195)	View Details	Edit
○	S6	rehabilitat*	Search modes - Boolean/Phrase	View Results (90,047)	View Details	Edit
○	S5	(MH "Rehabilitation+")	...ch modes - Boolean/Phrase	View Results (131,062)	View Details	Edit
○	S4	S2 OR S3	...Boolean/Phrase	View Results (41,870)	View Details	Edit
○	S3	stroke*	Sea... /Phrase	View Results (41,870)	View Details	Edit
○	S2	(MH "Stroke+")				Edit
○	S1	stroke AND rehabilitation				Edit

Different concepts combined with AND to give final result

Similar concept (Subject Term and free text) combined with OR

Viewing the results
Click on the 'View results' option to see the results. Only the title will be displayed and the publication type. To see more information, click on 'Page options' and select 'Detailed'.

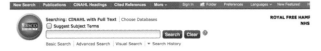

This will let you see the full citation, abstract, and subject terms. If full text is available, a link will appear beneath the record. Under 'Page options', you can also select the number of records per page that you want to see displayed.

Add to folder

To save citations, click on the 'Add to folder' link beneath each record. These results will automatically be saved until you are ready to print, export, email or save them.

To view the selected articles later, click on the 'Folder' link at the top of the screen. These will be lost once you log off, unless you create a personal account.

Personal account

You can set up a personal account, where you can save search strategies and results, and set up alerts, which let you know when new articles meeting your search criteria are added to the database. This feature is also available in other databases, including OVID and PubMed.

Saving search strategies

Once you have created your account, you can save your search strategies in your personal folder. To save searches, just click on Save Searches/Alerts, just above the search box, where you will also find links to Print Search History,

Retrieve Searches, and Retrieve Alerts. When you save a search, it is saved permanently, but you can also create an alert so that whenever a new paper is added to the database that meets your search criteria, then you will be automatically notified. This is a very useful feature for keeping up-to-date with the literature related to your search strategy.

Saving, printing, emailing or exporting records

You can either save/print/email/export each record, one at a time, or you can add them to your folder, and manage them all at the same time. Click on a record or go to your folder to see all your options.

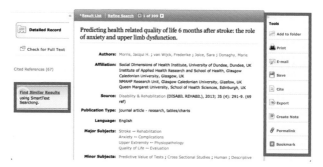

Find Similar Results

Another way to find potentially relevant articles in CINAHL is to use the 'Find Similar Results' feature. When you find a relevant citation from your search, click on the 'Find Similar Results' link to the left of the citation, and this will bring up a new list of articles that are 'related' (i.e. they have similar Subject Terms) to your chosen citation.

> If you wish to export citations from CINAHL into reference management software, you will need to select *Export*. This allows you to save your citations in a format which can be imported into a Citation Manager (see *Chapter 10: Saving citations*).

Cochrane Library (www.thecochranelibrary.com)

The Cochrane Library is a collection of databases that contain high-quality, independent evidence to inform healthcare decision-making. Cochrane reviews represent the highest level of evidence on which to base clinical treatment decisions. There are 53 Cochrane Review groups which publish systematic reviews. In addition to these reviews, there are systematic reviews from other providers, technology assessments, economic evaluations, and individual clinical trials. There are different levels of access, and more information can be found at: www.thecochranelibrary.com

	NOTE!
	For clinical searches, the Cochrane Library is a good place to start. However, bear in mind that you will retrieve less hits than other healthcare databases, because the content is mainly systematic reviews and randomised controlled trials, and restricted to the subjects covered by the Review Groups.

Scenario: A researcher is looking into methods for preventing the common cold and wants to know whether echinacea is more effective than vitamin C.

Focused question: *To prevent a common cold, is echinacea more effective than vitamin C?*

Problem	Intervention	Comparison	Outcome
common cold **OR** respiratory disorders	vitamin C **OR** ascorbic acid	echinacea	prevention

Type of question: Intervention/treatment or prevention
Best feasible study design: Systematic review or randomised controlled trial
Databases to search: Cochrane Library, CINAHL, Medline, Embase

Search process

Can I just type 'common cold AND vitamin C AND echinacea' into the main search box?
Yes, but this retrieves only one hit – do you think you have found everything?

You can improve your search using the search techniques we learned in Chapter 7: Free text and thesaurus searching.

Include a free text term and a MeSH for each relevant PICO term whenever possible.

There are three ways of searching the Cochrane Library: advanced search, MeSH search, and browse.

The 'advanced search' allows you to combine terms and apply limits, and lets you search via fields such as title and author. The 'MeSH search' gives you access to the thesaurus, and 'browse' lets you search through the topics. Search tips are available under the search box.

Advanced search

Think of all the alternate spellings for free text, and make use of truncation to expand word endings. The truncation symbol on the Cochrane Library is *. For example:

common cold OR respiratory disorder	Includes variations in terminology
nurse*	Finds nurse (singular) and nurses (plural)
nurs*	Finds nurse, nurses, nursing etc.
vitamin C OR ascorbic acid	Finds papers on vitamin C and ascorbic acid, which are the same thing

	NOTE!
	Be careful not to truncate too near the beginning of words, as you will retrieve too many alternatives.

The Cochrane Library allows you to search within fields so that you have some control over the results.

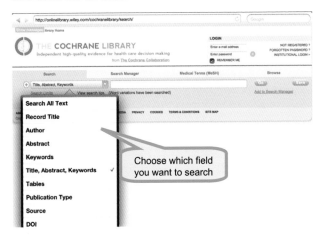

MeSH/Thesaurus

The Cochrane Library has a Thesaurus, a version of MeSH called 'Medical Terms'. Click on Advanced Search on the main page, choose the Medical Terms tab, enter a term, and click on Lookup. A list of terms, related to the search term entered will be displayed. The database will automatically explode the term, unless you select a tree or select Single MeSH term (unexploded).

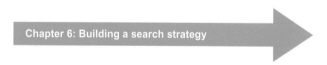

A summary of the search results, broken down by database will appear on the right-hand side, and there is the option to either save the search or add it to the Search Manager, where you will be able to combine with other terms.

Combining search terms

All searches are automatically stored in the Search History. From there, you can combine them using Boolean logic (AND, OR). Combine similar concepts with OR, different concepts with AND. More can be found on this concept in Chapter 6: Building a search strategy.

Chapter 6: Building a search strategy

Once you have all your search terms, go to the Search Manager tab and combine the searches as appropriate. An example of a search strategy is shown. Each line is numbered (e.g. #1, #2) – these line numbers should be used when combining searches.

Beneath the Search Manager box, there is the option to save searches. To do this you need to create an account, which you can freely do using the option in the top right-hand corner of the screen.

Limiting searches

Limits can only be applied in the Search tab, so if you want to apply limits to your search, then you need to combine Medical Terms and free text for the limits to work.

Viewing the results

In the Search History, the number of hits appears on the right-hand side of the search box.

To save results to file or reference management software choose Export.

Click on the number of hits to view the results, which are organised by database:

- Cochrane Reviews – this contains the full text and you need to click on the title to get access. They can be very comprehensive documents, so be careful when sending to print.
- Other Reviews – this is the Database of Reviews of Effects, and contains structured abstracts of systematic reviews, which have been assessed to ensure that the research has been carried out to the Cochrane Collaboration standards.
- Clinical Trials – CENTRAL is the most comprehensive source of abstracts of randomised controlled trials, collected from databases and using hand-searching techniques.
- Methods Studies – this contains studies of research methodologies.
- Technology Assessments – these are evaluations of whether the medical technology works, who it benefits, whether it is cost-effective, and how it compares with the alternatives.
- Economic Evaluations – this research looks at the cost-effectiveness of interventions.
- Cochrane Groups – there are 53 Cochrane Review Groups, and this database provides you with their contact details and further information of their work.

Click on the title to access the documents that you are interested in.

Saving, exporting or printing records
To save search results, use the Export facility, which lets you export the citations or citation and abstract into reference management software or to a text file. With the full text systematic reviews, you can save them individually as PDFs, or print them out. Cochrane Reviews can be very large documents and therefore need to be selected individually for printing.

Saving searches
To save a search strategy, you need to register for free with Wiley, the publishers of The Cochrane Library.

Alerts
The alerts function allows you to receive email updates related to your search strategy, so that each time an article matching your search criteria is added to the database, an email is sent to you, notifying you of the new addition. This service is free, although you do need to register to use it.

User guides
The Cochrane Library has help available, in a range of different languages. Visit the help page for more information. A useful resource is the *Cochrane Handbook*,[11] as this explains the processes for carrying out a systematic literature search.

Further reading
Crumley, E.T., Wiebe, N., Cramer, K., Klassen, T.P. & Hartling, L. 2005. Which resources should be used to identify RCT/CCTs for systematic reviews: a systematic review. *BMC Med Res Methodol*, 5, 24 available from: PM:16092960
✓**Full text:** www.biomedcentral.com/1471-2288/5/24/

Wilkins, T., Gillies, R.A. & Davies, K. 2005. EMBASE versus MEDLINE for family medicine searches: can MEDLINE searches find the forest or a tree? *Can Fam Physician*, 51, 848–849 available from: PM:16926954
✓**Full text:** www.ncbi.nlm.nih.gov/pmc/articles/PMC1479531/

---

[11] Higgins, J.P.T., Green, S. Eds. Updated March 2011. *Cochrane Handbook for Systematic Reviews of Interventions Version 5.1.0*. The Cochrane Collaboration available from www.cochrane-handbook.org.

CHAPTER 9
Refining search results

If your search strategy has retrieved too many results, you might like to refine your search using limits or search filters. Both can be applied at the start of the search process or at the end.

Limits

Once your search has been completed, many databases allow you to 'Limit' the results using specific Fields. Applying limits reduces the amount of hits by retrieving only those records matching the chosen limit/s.

A Field is a specific structural unit of a database record, like Title or Author.

Common fields to limit by include:

Language (.la)	Although a journal article might be in a language other than English, an English abstract is usually included, so be wary about limiting by language.
Age	The major healthcare databases vary in age limits: • <u>CINAHL</u> – conception to approx 6 months after delivery, conception to birth, up to one month old, 1–23 months, 2–5 years, 6–12 years, 13–18 years, 19–44 years, 45–64 years, 65–79 years, 80+ years • <u>Embase</u> – adults, older people, all children, children, infants, preschool children, school-age children, adolescents • <u>Medline</u> – all adults, adults – 19 and over, 19–44 years, 45–64 years, 65–79 years, 80 and over, all children – 0–18 years, all infants birth to 23 months, birth to 1 month, 1–23 months, 2–12 years, 2–5 years, 6–12 years, 13–18 years • <u>PsycINFO</u> – birth to 12 years, birth to one month, 2–23 months, 2–5 years, 6–12 years, 13–17 years, 18 years and older, 18–29 years, 30–39 years, 40–64 years, 65 years and older, 85 years and older
Title (.ti)	Looks for your keywords only in the Title of an article – this is restrictive and will miss much relevant information, but usually retrieves very relevant articles
Publication Year(.py)	Retrieves all articles published in one year, or a range of years
Author (.au)	Use when searching for articles by a specific author(s)

Searching Skills Toolkit: Finding the Evidence, Second Edition. Caroline De Brún and Nicola Pearce-Smith.
© 2014 John Wiley & Sons, Ltd. Published 2014 by John Wiley & Sons, Ltd.

Worked example (OvidSP Medline)

A search limited by English language and the publication years 2010–2012:

Further options to limit can be obtained by clicking on 'Additional Limits'. Other limits include:

- Humans or Animals
- Publication Types (see next section) – as with the age groups, the major healthcare databases differ in the types of publication they offer.

Worked example (PubMed)

A search limited by English Language, published in the last 3 years and specific to Humans:

Publication types

Limiting by attributes such as Date or Language is possible as shown, but it is not the best way to limit your search if you are interested in finding better quality research studies.

Another way to limit your search is to use the Publication Type field, as this allows you to search for particular study types such as:

- Meta-Analysis
- Randomised Controlled Trial
- Clinical Trial
- Practice Guideline.

For example, if you have a Treatment/Intervention question, limit your search using the Meta-Analysis or Randomised Controlled Trial Article types on PubMed.

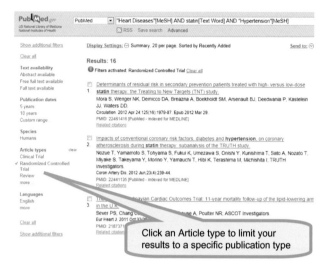

Applying limits within your search strategy

Limits may also be applied during your search, by typing the specific field name after your search term.

	Ovid	PubMed	EBSCO
looks for the word 'hypertension' in the **title**	hypertension.ti	hypertension[ti]	TI hypertension
looks for records with the word 'statin' in the **title or abstract**	statin.tw. or statin.ti,ab	statin[tiab]	TI statin or AB statin
looks for records with 'BMJ' in the **journal title**	BMJ.jn	BMJ[ta]	JT BMJ

Methodological filters

A methodological search filter is a search strategy containing search terms that relate to a research methodology (i.e. the study design). The search terms may be thesaurus (e.g. MeSH), free text, publication types or a combination of all three. A filter can be used to retrieve articles of appropriate study design, to answer a particular type of question.

> You may see search filters described as:
> - 'hedges'
> - optimal search strategies
> - research methodology filters
> - Clinical Queries.

A search filter may just be one or two search terms – see the following table. You can combine these single filter terms with your subject search, to assist you in finding appropriate study designs.

Question type	Best feasible study design	Best single Medline search term
DIAGNOSIS	Cross-sectional study	Sensitivity
HARM	Cohort study	Risk
PROGNOSIS	Cohort study	Explode Cohort Studies [MeSH]
TREATMENT	Systematic review or randomised controlled trial	Meta-analysis(pt) or Randomised Controlled Trial(pt)

Table adapted from Users' Guides to the Medical Literature.[12]

> *MeSH = Medical Subject Heading*
> *pt = Publication Type*
> *Explode = inclusion of all narrower MeSH*

Worked example (Ovid Medline)
What is the risk of type II diabetes for adults who are obese and take little exercise? Type of question: HARM

---

[12] Guyatt, G., Drummond, R. 2002. *Users' Guides to the Medical Literature: Essentials of Evidence-based Clinical Practice.* American Medical Association, Chicago.

Clinical Queries

There are comprehensive, validated methodological search filters available for use, developed by Haynes et al.[10] These filters can be applied to your searches in Medline (using PubMed, Ovid or Dialog) – they are known as *Clinical Queries*.

The filters contain search terms (including publication types and free text words) designed to retrieve particular clinical study types. There are categories for aetiology (harm), diagnosis, therapy and prognosis, corresponding to the four main types of clinical question.

To see details about the search strategies that make up these filters, go to PubMed Clinical Queries and click on 'filter information': www.ncbi.nlm.nih.gov/pubmed/clinical

Worked example (PubMed)

Click on 'Clinical Queries' from PubMed homepage.

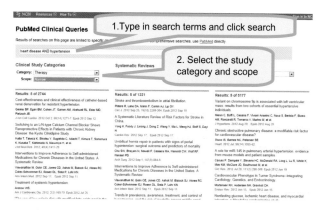

Sensitivity versus specificity

The terms 'sensitivity' and 'specificity' each have two meanings in evidence-based healthcare – one for statistics and one for searching. The application of sensitivity and specificity filters when searching is another way of refining your search.

The use of these terms in statistics refers to the accuracy of a diagnostic test. In the case of statistics, 'sensitivity' refers to how good a test is at correctly identifying people who have the disease, while 'specificity' is more concerned with how good the test is at correctly identifying people who are well.[13] Ideally, they should both be 100%, but this is rarely the case.

In the context of searching, the terms again apply to accuracy, but this time in terms of number of results retrieved. You can perform a 'sensitive (broad)' or a 'specific (narrow)' search when using Clinical Queries. On PubMed this is called the Scope.

Sensitivity = high recall, low precision (i.e. retrieves more of the relevant articles, but at the expense of picking up more unwanted articles).

Specificity = lower recall, higher precision (i.e. more of the articles retrieved will be relevant (proportionally), but some of the relevant articles may be missed).

---

[13]Loong, T.W. 2003. Understanding sensitivity and specificity with the right side of the brain. *BMJ*, 327(7417), 716–719 available from www.bmj.com/cgi/content/full/327/7417/716.

For example, a **sensitive** search may pick up 200 of the 225 relevant articles on your topic in Medline but will also retrieve 500 irrelevant articles (total recall of 700). A **specific** search may pick up only 100 of the relevant 225 articles in Medline, but will only retrieve 50 irrelevant articles (total recall of 150).

When using Clinical Queries, a sensitive search will retrieve a greater number of the available articles of relevant study design, but will also pick up many unwanted articles. Proportionally, more of the articles retrieved in a specific search will be of a relevant study design, but some available relevant articles will be missed.

Worked example (Ovid Medline)

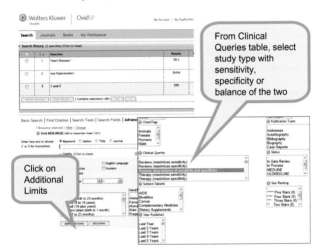

From Clinical Queries table, select study type with sensitivity, specificity or balance of the two

Click on Additional Limits

Clinical Queries filters only search the Medline content. There are other clinical databases where you will find relevant research, and although there is some overlap, there will also be new content on these databases. You can read more about other clinical databases in Chapter 3: Clinical information: sources.

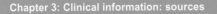

Chapter 3: Clinical information: sources

Some of these databases will also have inbuilt filters, but for those that do not, you will have to construct your own searches. This is easily done, as many filters are widely available on the Internet. Just type in the terms that they have used and save the search so that you can use it again. Here are some resources:

- Clinical Queries:
   www.ncbi.nlm.nih.gov/pubmed/clinical click on 'filter information'
- InterTASC Information Specialists' Sub-Group Search Filter Resource
   www.york.ac.uk/inst/crd/intertasc/index.htm
- Scottish Intercollegiate Guidelines Network
   www.sign.ac.uk/methodology/filters.html

For more help, contact your local medical librarian or use the database help pages.

How do I do know whether to conduct a specific or sensitive search?

This depends on factors such as how much time you have, the reason you are doing the search and how much evidence there is on your topic. Choosing to conduct a sensitive search will mean the search will be more inclusive – you are less likely to miss something relevant, but you will need more time to look through the results for relevance.

Conversely, the results from a specific search will take less time to look through and many will be relevant, but you have to accept that you won't have retrieved all the relevant articles – you may wish to use a specific search to quickly find articles of appropriate study design for use in immediate patient care.

Systematic reviews

There are several important databases containing systematic reviews, including the Cochrane Library and DARE – see Chapter 3: Clinical information: sources.

Chapter 3: Clinical information: sources

Medline also indexes systematic reviews, including Cochrane reviews, and these can be quickly found by using the Clinical Queries search box in PubMed.

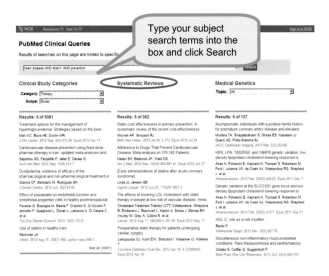

Note that this PubMed systematic review filter also retrieves those articles indexed as meta-analyses, reviews of clinical trials, evidence-based medicine, consensus development conferences and guidelines.

Further reading

Agoritsas, T., Merglen, A., Courvoisier, D.S., Combescure, C., Garin, N., Perrier, A. & Perneger, T.V. 2012. Sensitivity and predictive value of 15 PubMed search strategies to answer clinical questions rated against full systematic reviews. *J Med Internet Res*, 14(3), e85 available from: PM:22693047
✓**Full text:** www.jmir.org/2012/3/e85/

Fraser, C., Murray, A. & Burr, J. 2006. Identifying observational studies of surgical interventions in MEDLINE and EMBASE. *BMC Med Res Methodol*, 6, 41 available from: PM:16919159
✓**Full text:** www.biomedcentral.com/1471-2288/6/41

Glanville, J., Bayliss, S., Booth, A., et al. 2008. So many filters, so little time: the development of a search filter appraisal checklist. *J Med Libr Assoc*, 96(4), 356–361 available from: PM:18974813
✓**Full text:** www.ncbi.nlm.nih.gov/pmc/articles/PMC2568852/

Golder, S. & Loke, Y.K. 2012. The performance of adverse effects search filters in MEDLINE and EMBASE. *Health Info Libr J*, 29(2), 141–151 available from: PM:22630362

Golder, S., McIntosh, H.M. & Loke, Y. 2006. Identifying systematic reviews of the adverse effects of healthcare interventions. *BMC Med Res Methodol*, 6, 22 available from: PM:16681854
✓**Full text:** www.ncbi.nlm.nih.gov/pmc/articles/PMC1481562/

Kable, A.K., Pich, J. & Maslin-Prothero, S.E. 2012. A structured approach to documenting a search strategy for publication: a 12 step guideline for authors. *Nurse Educ Today* available from: PM:22633885

Haase, A., Follmann, M., Skipka, G. & Kirchner, H. 2007. Developing search strategies for clinical practice guidelines in SUMSearch and Google Scholar and assessing their retrieval performance. *BMC Med Res Methodol*, 7, 28 available from: PM:17603909
✓**Full text:** www.ncbi.nlm.nih.gov/pmc/articles/PMC1925105/

Haynes, R.B., Kastner, M. & Wilczynski, N.L. 2005. Developing optimal search strategies for detecting clinically sound and relevant causation studies in EMBASE. *BMC Med Inform Decis Mak*, 5, 8 available from: PM:15784134
✓**Full text:** www.biomedcentral.com/1472-6947/5/8

Hempel, S., Rubenstein, L.V., Shanman, R.M., Foy, R., Golder, S., Danz, M. & Shekelle, P.G. 2011. Identifying quality improvement intervention publications – a comparison of electronic search strategies. *Implement Sci*, 6, 85 available from: PM:21806808
✓**Full text:** www.rrsstq.com/stock/fra/publications/P200.pdf

Kastner, M., Wilczynski, N.L., Walker-Dilks, C., McKibbon, K.A. & Haynes, B. 2006. Age-specific search strategies for Medline. *J Med Internet Res*, 8(4), e25 available from: PM:17213044
✓**Full text:** www.jmir.org/2006/4/e25/

Lee, E., Dobbins, M., Decorby, K., McRae, L., Tirilis, D. & Husson, H. 2012. An optimal search filter for retrieving systematic reviews and meta-analyses. *BMC Med Res Methodol*, 12(1), 51 available from: PM:22512835
✓**Full text:** www.biomedcentral.com/1471-2288/12/51/abstract

Motschall, E., Anntes, G. & Klar, R. 2002. Efficient Medline search filters for clinical queries. Institute of Medical Biometrics and Medical Informatics, Freiburg, Germany
✓**Full text:** www.opac.zbmed.de/fileadmin/pdf_dateien/EAHIL_2002/motschall-proc.pdf

Sampson, M., Zhang, L., Morrison, A., Barrowman, N.J., Clifford, T.J., Platt, R.W., Klassen, T.P. & Moher, D. 2006. An alternative to the hand searching gold standard: validating methodological search filters using relative recall. *BMC Med Res Methodol*, 6, 33 available from: PM:16848895
✓**Full text:** www.ncbi.nlm.nih.gov/pmc/articles/PMC1557524/

Sandars, S. & Del Mar, C. 2005. Editorial: Clever searching for evidence: new search filters can help to find the needle in the haystack. *BMJ*, 330(7501), 1162–1163 available from: PM:15905232

Van, W.C., Bennett, C. & Forster, A.J. 2010. Derivation and validation of a MEDLINE search strategy for research studies that use administrative data. *Health Serv.Res*, 45(6 Pt 1), 1836–1845 available from: PM:20819111

CHAPTER 10
Saving citations

Scenario: You perform a search using PubMed Clinical Queries, and feel pleased with yourself as you find a systematic review that helps you to treat a specific patient. Six months later, the same treatment question crops up again for a different patient, but you can't remember what the paper was or where you found it, so you have to do the search again.

Does this sound familiar?

Here are two ways that you can record or save details about useful papers you find from your searches, so that you can retrieve them at a later date.

Logbooks

Jot down clinical questions when they arise, and if you have a chance to search for papers to answer some of them, write down your search terms, the citation/s and a summary of their results, for example the clinical bottom line.

An example of how this might look:

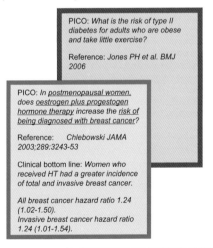

PICO: *What is the risk of type II diabetes for adults who are obese and take little exercise?*

Reference: *Jones PH et al. BMJ 2006*

PICO: *In postmenopausal women, does oestrogen plus progestogen hormone therapy increase the risk of being diagnosed with breast cancer?*

Reference: *Chlebowski JAMA 2003;289:3243-53*

Clinical bottom line: *Women who received HT had a greater incidence of total and invasive breast cancer.*

All breast cancer hazard ratio 1.24 (1.02-1.50).
Invasive breast cancer hazard ratio 1.24 (1.01-1.54).

Searching Skills Toolkit: Finding the Evidence, Second Edition. Caroline De Brún and Nicola Pearce-Smith.
© 2014 John Wiley & Sons, Ltd. Published 2014 by John Wiley & Sons, Ltd.

You can develop a template in Word or even collect your clinical questions using mobile technologies, such as smartphones or tablets.

Reference management software

There are also software packages, or 'citation managers', that enable you to save details of useful citations.

> You may see software for saving, managing and publishing citations described as:
> *Citation managers*
> *Citation management software*
> *Bibliographic management software*
> *Bibliographic publishing tools*
> *Reference management software.*

Citation managers allow you to export references directly from databases (e.g. Medline) or from some web pages (e.g. electronic journals like *BMJ*, *JAMA*). You can also add references manually, search, create a bibliography and 'cite while you write' (facility to add citations to a document you are writing).

Subscription only

Subscription only citation managers include:
- Procite
  www.procite.com
- Reference Manager
  www.refman.com
- EndNote
  www.endnote.com
- RefWorks
  www.refworks.com

All of these packages have similar features – most of them allow you to download a free trial before making a purchase.

Freely available

Freely available citation managers include:
- Mendeley
  www.mendeley.com
- Zotero
  www.zotero.com

Both of these packages have similar features and are free to download.

This example from Ovid Medline shows the Direct Export of citations. After selecting the articles you wish to keep, click on Export to open the Export Citation list.

Choose appropriate citation manager to export your references

The example here shows an EndNote database after citations have been imported.

EndNote

MENDELEY

Mendeley (www.mendeley.com/)
Mendeley is free reference management software and it lets you import citations in three ways:
1. directly from the online databases
2. manual import, one at a time by adding or drag-and-drop method
3. web importer which sits on your browser.

Once imported, they can be organised into folders, which is very useful, particularly, if you are researching different clinical topics, because you can keep them all separate, but stored in one place. Mendeley is available to download to your home computer and via the Internet, and there are also iPad and iPhone apps available.

You can add the original documents in Word or PDF, and then store them on your home/work computer, while making the citations available on any computer/tablet/smartphone via the Internet version of Mendeley. It is also possible to read and annotate PDFs, highlighting key statements.

As with Endnote, Mendeley has a cite-while-you-write feature that allows you to add citations to reports and papers that you are writing, and automatically creates bibliographies in the reference management style of your choice. Tutorials are available on the site to help you learn how to use the site, although it is fairly intuitive.

Individual citation

Organise papers into folders

List of all the papers that you are reading

zotero

Zotero (www.zotero.org/)

Like Mendeley, this is a freely-available resource to help you collect, organise, cite and share citations. It has a desktop version and an Internet version, and allows you to add references manually, as a batch from databases. It also has unique one-click import functionality.

Cite while you write

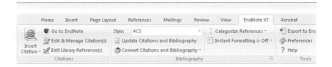

Another clever thing that citation managers can do is to enable you to 'cite while you write'. This allows you to access and easily cite references in Microsoft Word (shown here), and create a document with formatted references and a bibliography.

CHAPTER 11
Citation pearl searching

Sometimes when you have run your search, the results may not be exactly what you are looking for. Out of 50 results, for example, only one may be relevant. So what do you do next?

Option 1
Give up and end up none the wiser.

Option 2
Investigate further and find the pearl!

Option 2 is 'citation pearl searching' or 'citation pearl growing'.[14] This method means taking the few results that you do have and using them to identify more relevant papers. There are a number of ways to do this.

Related items

Many databases and search engines now identify 'related items' or 'similar items' that could be what you are looking for, for example, 'Related citations in PubMed':

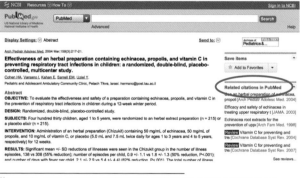

---

[14]Ramer, S.L. 2005. Site-ation pearl growing: methods and librarianship history and theory. *Journal of the Medical Library Association*, 93(3), 397–400.

In the example, a relevant article looking at the use of vitamin C as a means of relieving the symptoms of the common cold was retrieved. Only 27 results were found, and the one displayed was the most relevant. On the right of the screen, however, 'Related citations' are identified, which did not appear in the original search, but which might be relevant. It would be a good idea to look at those records and see whether they are using terms that you have not included in your search strategy, and then adding such terms to your strategy.

Similarly, Google Scholar has 'Related articles', BMJ and JAMA have 'Related Content':

Author search

It is possible to search using an author's surname and initials to see what else they have written. Many journal websites already have links, such as 'Articles by [author name]' so that you can see whether they have written more papers on the same topic. On PubMed, this is very easy because the author names are hyperlinked, so just click on the author name and you are taken to other research by this author. This feature is available in many databases and electronic journals.

Another option is to contact the authors directly to see whether they have written (or indeed are writing) anything else on this topic or whether they know of any other researchers who have written on the same topic. Nowadays, many journals will publish author contact details to facilitate collaboration.

Keywords

After performing a search, if you only find one good and relevant reference, go into the full record and look at the keywords / thesaurus terms / MeSH terms / descriptors etc. to see whether they have been indexed using terms you have not included in your search. Sometimes, different languages and databases apply alternative terminology. For example, the Medline and CINAHL index's use the MeSH term 'Emergency Medical Technicians', while

Embase uses 'Paramedical Personnel' for paramedic. If you do not include all the relevant terms in your search, then you might miss out on key research.

In PubMed, if you change the Display settings to Medline, the list of MeSH or descriptors headings will be shown:

```
 MH    Aged
 MH   - Antiviral Agents/therapeutic use
 MH   - Ascorbic Acid/therapeutic use
 MH   - Common Cold/*therapy
 MH   - *Echinacea
 MH   - Female
 MH   - Humans
 MH   - Male
 MH   - Middle Aged
 MH   - Oxadiazoles/therapeutic use
 MH   - Phytotherapy
 MH   - Plant Extracts/therapeutic use
 MH   - Questionnaires
 MH   - Risk Assessment
 MH   - Severity of Illness Index
 MH   - Treatment Outcome
 MH   - Vitamins/therapeutic use
 MH   - Zinc Compounds/therapeutic use
 EDAT- 2007/06/06 09:00
 MHDA- 2007/08/01 09:00
```

Journals

Many journals, including the *British Medical Journal*, *The Journal of the American Medical Association*, *New England Journal of Medicine*, and *the Lancet*, offer a range of methods for citation pearl searching, including 'Find similar articles in PubMed' on the *BMJ* site and 'Articles Related by Topic' on the *JAMA* site.

Snowballing

One final place to search for similar papers is in the list of references supplied by the author at the end of the relevant article. Often this is a good place to look when searching for similar titles or authors who are looking at the same topics. Particularly with online papers, the individual references may even hyperlink straight to the original papers. By looking at the references that they have used, you can also identify additional terminology that can be added to the search strategy.[15]

---

[15] Greenhalgh, T., Peacock, R. 2005 Effectiveness and efficiency of search methods in systematic reviews of complex evidence: audit of primary sources. *BMJ*. 331(7524), 1064.

Alerts

Journals often provide alerting services, such as when it is cited, when responses are posted and when a correction is posted, so that you can keep up to date with any developments related to the original article. This is a useful way to stay current with any changes in your field of research.

RSS feeds

 RSS feeds are a way of receiving information and keeping up to date. Many websites are providing RSS feeds and you can recognise them with symbols similar to this one or with RSS or XML in white with an orange background. To read the feeds you need to set up a page on a news reader or an aggregator, such as NetVibes or Hootsuite. Internet browsers often let you collect RSS feeds like favourites, and Microsoft Outlook lets you store RSS feeds alongside your emails, in a separate folder. These resources will collect all of your RSS feeds. Every time your favourite websites are updated, they will automatically send details to your news reader. This means that instead of visiting lots of websites to see whether there is any new content, you can just go to one and see all the updates in one place. RSS feeds are particularly useful for journal content pages and search results so that each time new research is added to the database that meets with your search criteria, you will automatically be alerted to this. A useful tutorial on RSS is available from Common Craft www.commoncraft.com/rss_plain_english

 It is worth making a note of the methods that you use, in case you need to write up your literature review, and also to ensure that you don't get lost!

CHAPTER 12

Quality improvement and value: sources

Searching for information on commissioning, quality improvement, and cost is important for management decision-making, particularly during these times of recession, when people and organisations are being asked to do more with less. It is essential that evidence-based principles are applied to management and policy decisions. The emphasis in healthcare at the moment is on efficiency and value for money, whilst improving the quality of services and treatments available. Searching for information on these topics is not always easy, because:

- subjects may cut across all clinical disciplines
- search terms may be very diverse, not well defined, or relatively new
- resources that contain such information are not always indexed on standard databases like Medline or Embase.

Examples of quality improvement and value questions

1. Can we reduce the cost and improve the quality of care for cancer patients?
2. How can we be cost-effective in treating diabetes patients in primary care?
3. Can we safely reduce the current level of medical pre-operative testing before surgery?
4. How can the ward be cleaned effectively, whilst keeping the costs down?
5. How can lean processes improve practice in primary care?
6. How many services are there for people with musculoskeletal disease in the North West, and which gives best value?
7. How does our service for children with mental health problems compare with other regions?

There are a number of sources of high quality information which provide the evidence base, and this section will highlight key resources and suggest appropriate search terms to identify relevant evidence.

Current awareness

A quick way to stay up to date on cost and quality topics is via relevant blogs and newsletters; some examples are given here:

Searching Skills Toolkit: Finding the Evidence, Second Edition. Caroline De Brún and Nicola Pearce-Smith.
© 2014 John Wiley & Sons, Ltd. Published 2014 by John Wiley & Sons, Ltd.

- QIPP @lert
  www.qippalert.blogspot.com/
- NHS Right Care @lert
  www.rightcare.nhs.uk
- King's Fund alert service
  www.kingsfund.org.uk
- Commissioning Elf
  www.thecommissioningelf.net/
- Chair on Knowledge Transfer and Innovation in Canada e-watch newsletter
  www.santepop.qc.ca/en/

Searching for evidence on quality improvement and value

Searching for evidence about quality, in particular, can be difficult because there are so many terms which could be considered for inclusion. Also, some subject headings, like 'Quality Improvement' retrieve several thousand hits, so must be combined with a subject/topic to restrict the search. Here we have listed some subject headings and free text terms which we have found useful when searching databases for information on quality improvement, commissioning or value in healthcare. See Chapter 7: Free text and thesaurus searching for more guidance. It is not a comprehensive list, and there are not yet many specific index terms; for example there is currently no subject heading for 'value' in the context of value for money/best value, or for

Subject headings	Free text
Accountable care organizations	accountable care
Cost benefit analysis	best value
Cost control	better value
Cost effectiveness analysis	commissioning
Cost savings	disinvestment
Costs and cost analysis	high* value
Delivery of healthcare, integrated	low* value
Economic evaluation	prioriti?ation
Efficiency	priority setting
Efficiency audit	program* budgeting
Efficiency improvement	quality improv*
Efficiency, organizational	unwarranted variation
Healthcare costs	waste
Healthcare quality	
Healthcare rationing	
Health priorities	
Outcome assessment (healthcare)	
Productivity	
Quality improvement	

'commissioning'. As terms like this become more widely used, new subject headings terms may be added to database indexes to reflect this.

If you have a relevant article already, or find one from a search, it may be useful to try 'citation pearl searching', using Related Citations on PubMed or other methods. This enables you to identify other relevant articles which you may have missed when searching. It also allows you to discover other useful search terms, especially from the abstract, which can be incorporated into a new search.

Chapter 11: Citation pearl searching

As well as standard medical databases like Medline, you should also try searching databases such as:

- EconLit – citations to international publications on economics, available via Ovid (subscription required)
- Health Business Elite – healthcare administration and management citations, available via EBSCO (subscription required)
- Health Management Information Consortium (HMIC) – containing health and social care management and services information, available via Ovid (subscription required)
- Health Technology Assessment (HTA) – ongoing and completed health technology assessments from around the world
  www.crd.york.ac.uk/crdweb/
- McMaster University Health Systems Evidence – syntheses of research evidence about governance, financial and delivery arrangements within health systems
  www.mcmasterhealthforum.org/healthsystemsevidence-en
- NHS Economic Evaluation Database (NHS EED) – economic evaluations of healthcare interventions
  www.crd.york.ac.uk/crdweb/
- PDQ-Evidence for Informed Health Policymaking – best evidence for informing decisions about health systems
  www.pdq-evidence.org/
- PubMed Comparative Effectiveness Reviews – published research to help inform investigations of comparative effectiveness
  www.nlm.nih.gov/nichsr/cer/cerqueries.html
- The Cochrane Effective Practice and Organisation of Care Group (EPOC) – reviews of interventions designed to improve professional practice and the delivery of effective health services
  www.epoc.cochrane.org/

Other useful sources of information

Luckily, you may find that information on the quality and value of
healthcare services has been found and collated for you already. There are
NHS and other reputable organisations that provide resources, alerts and
tools useful for these topics. We have highlighted some of our
recommended ones.

NHS England (formerly the NHS Commissioning Board)
(www.england.nhs.uk/)

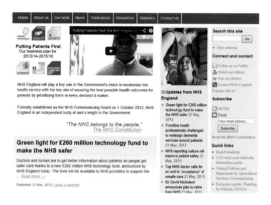

The main aim of NHS England is to improve the health outcomes for people
in England.

It was responsible for the authorisation of the 211 clinical commissioning
groups (CCGs), which are the drivers of the new, clinically-led commissioning
system. NHS England has now taken on many of the functions of the former
primary care trusts, as well as some nationally-based functions previously
undertaken by the Department of Health.

Areas of work include direct commissioning, quality improvement and
clinical leadership, governing frameworks and patient safety. As part of NHS
England, an improvement organisation has been created to bring together
health knowledge and expertise – NHS Improving Quality (NHS IQ)
www.nhsiq.nhs.uk/. NHS IQ will draw on the experience of previous
improvement programmes such as NHS Improvement and the NHS Institute
for Innovation and Improvement, which are now closed.

The site contains bulletins, blogs, factsheets, frameworks, commissioning
information, tools, statistics and resources for CCGs, senates and
commissioning support units.

NICE – Quality, Innovation, Productivity and Prevention (QIPP) (www.evidence.nhs.uk/qipp/)

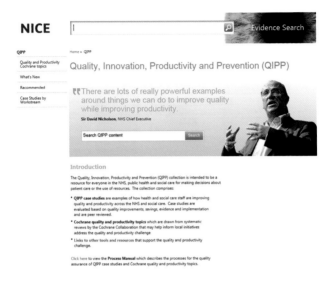

The QIPP collection is an NHS resource for making decisions about patient care and the use of resources.

The collection contains QIPP case studies – examples of how staff are improving quality and productivity across the NHS and social care; Cochrane quality and productivity topics – (systematic reviews by the Cochrane Collaboration, that may help to address the quality and productivity challenge), and links to tools and resources.

NICE commissioning guides

(www.nice.org.uk/usingguidance/commissioningguides/bytopic.jsp)

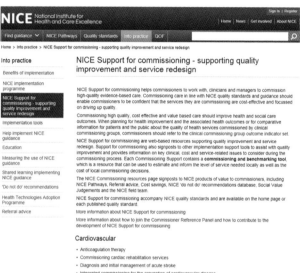

NICE provides guidance to ensure quality and value for money in healthcare.
These commissioning guides contain a commissioning and benchmarking tool, which is a resource that can be used to estimate and inform the level of service needed locally as well as the cost of local commissioning decisions.

In addition to the Commissioning Guides, NICE also produce Quality Standards, designed to operate alongside guidelines, to drive quality improvements within a particular area of healthcare. These are available here: www.nice.org.uk/guidance/qualitystandards/qualitystandards.jsp.

Right Care (www.rightcare.nhs.uk/)

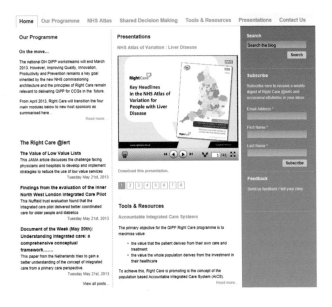

Right Care is a Department of Health Quality, Innovation, Productivity and Prevention (QIPP) workstream, whose aim is to maximise value to the patient and to the whole population.

Many resources are available on their website, including presentations, tools and an alert service.

The Right Care website provides access to Casebooks (local examples of commissioning work), Essential Reading (a series of reading lists on themes such as value, disinvestment and integrated care), and tools (such as the Clinical Commissioning Group Spend and Outcomes Tool). Right Care also produces the *NHS Atlas of Variation*, and other themed atlases, to support the search for unexplained variations and help clinicians to see where to focus their attention to improve the care they provide.

Although the Right Care project finished in April 2013, all existing products of Right Care will remain accessible from the Right Care website until further notice, and these outputs will remain accessible to the NHS into the future.

The Nuffield Trust (www.nuffieldtrust.org.uk/)

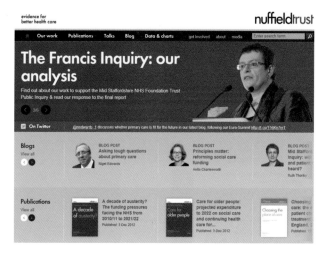

The Nuffield Trust is an independent source of evidence-based research and policy analysis for improving healthcare in the UK.

They produce reports, blogs and interactive data on topics such as commissioning, competition and provision of care.

The King's Fund (www.kingsfund.org.uk/)

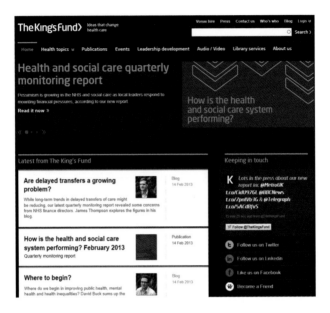

The King's Fund is an independent charity working to improve health and social care in England.

They produce reports, blogs, literature searches and an online database covering topics such as commissioning, productivity and finance, quality of care and integrated care.

Health Foundation (www.health.org.uk/)

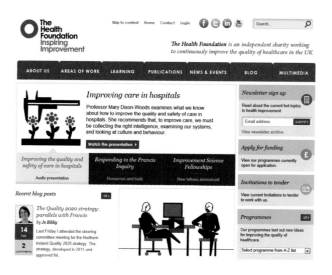

The Health Foundation is an independent charity working to improve the quality of healthcare.

They provide publications, blogs and the latest research on quality, safety and shared decision-making in healthcare.

Healthcare Quality Improvement Partnership (HQIP)
(www.hqip.org.uk/)

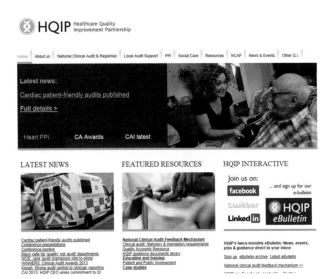

HQIP promotes quality in healthcare, and aims to increase the impact that clinical audit has on healthcare quality in England and Wales. HQIP has information on local and national clinical audits, patient and public involvement and social care.

There are many other organisations around the world publishing research on related topics such as health management and service improvement. Many have newsletters so that you can be informed by email when new research has been published.

- Agency for Healthcare Research and Quality
  www.ahrq.gov/research/findings/factsheets/costs/costix.html
- Audit Commission
  www.audit-commission.gov.uk/
- Canadian Foundation for Healthcare Improvement
  www.cfhi-fcass.ca/
- The Change Foundation
  www.changefoundation.ca/

- Improvement And Development Agency (IDEA)
    www.local.gov.uk/
- Institute for Health Improvement
    www.ihi.org/
- NESTA (National Endowment for Science, Technology and the Arts)
    www.nesta.org.uk/
- NHS Confederation
    www.nhsconfed.org/
- Picker Institute
    www.pickereurope.org/

A number of universities have their own health economics centres, where they publish their research. Some examples are given here:
- University of Birmingham Health Services Research Centre
    www.birmingham.ac.uk/schools/social-policy/departments/
    health-services-management-centre/
- University of Oxford Health Economics Research Centre
    www.herc.ox.ac.uk/research
- University of York Centre for Health Economics
    www.york.ac.uk/che/

Networks

Sharing good practice is an important part of improving service delivery. Here are a few relevant networks:
- Commissioning Zone – contains discussion lists and newsfeeds to support commissioners
    www.networks.nhs.uk/commissioning
- CHAIN – online support network for people working in health and social care
    www.chain.ulcc.ac.uk/chain/index.html
- NHS Networks – provides a common space for NHS staff to explore ideas, pool experience, solve problems and share information
    www.networks.nhs.uk/
- Knowledge 4 Commissioning – provides evidence services and case studies to commissioning organisations
    www.knowledge4commissioning.nhs.uk/

Keep a list of 'Favourites' on your Internet browser, so you can easily find all these websites, and add other useful websites that you come across. Also, make sure you store details of any relevant publications or articles you find, using one of the techniques outlined in Chapter 10: Saving citations.

Chapter 10: Saving citations

Further reading

Evans,B.A., Snooks, H., Howson, H. & Davies, M. 2013. How hard can it be to include research evidence and evaluation in local health policy implementation? Results from a mixed methods study. *Implementation Science*, 8:17
✓**Full text:** www.implementationscience.com/content/pdf/1748-5908-8-17.pdf

Fan, E., Laupacis, A., Pronovost, P.J., Guyatt, G.H. & Needham, D.M. 2010. How to use an article about quality improvement. *JAMA*, 304(20), 2279–2287 available from: PM:21098772
✓**Full text:** www.mhakeystonecenter.org/documents/january2011/tab_iiie_2279.pdf

Moat, K.A., Lavis, Wilson, M.G., Rottingen, J-A. & Barnighausen, T. 2013. Twelve myths about systematic reviews for health system policymaking rebutted. *Journal of Health Services Research & Policy*, 18(1), 44–50 available from: PMID: 23393042
✓**Full text:** www.jhsrp.rsmjournals.com/content/18/1/44.full.pdf+html

Phillips, C. 2009. What is cost-effectiveness? 2nd ed. Hayward Medical Communications, London
✓**Full text:** www.medicine.ox.ac.uk/bandolier/painres/download/whatis/Cost-effect.pdf

White, R. 2010. NHS 'quality' initiatives: acronyms and terminology. *Wounds UK*, 6(1), 155
✓**Full text:** www.wounds-uk.com/pdf/content_9354.pdf

CHAPTER 13
Patient information: sources

Consumer health information is reliable healthcare evidence that has been adapted for use by the lay person, and can help patients and carers make an informed decision about some aspect of their health.

With the growth in technology and increased access to online health information of variable quality, there is a greater need for skills in information literacy, particularly with regards to health information. While people have computer access, they often do not have the skills to find and assess the information that they need. This chapter is designed to help health professionals, patients and carers find good quality, online consumer health information. It highlights some of the tools, decision aids, and resources designed for and available to patients.

Shared decision-making

Shared decision-making is very high on the government agenda at the

moment as it benefits the patient and the health organisation in terms of well-being, service improvement, and cost-efficiency.

Evidence shows[16] that when people are involved in the decision made about their treatment choice, they are more likely to comply with the treatment regime,
because they have a greater understanding of what is involved. Yet to make an informed choice, as with health professionals, patients need to have the best available information, and this is where the issues lie. Health professionals have access to medical libraries, populated with appropriate resources and staff to support evidence-based practice or informed decision-making. Patients rarely have access to medical libraries, and the Internet is often their most easily accessible option for obtaining information. During consultations, doctors may not have the time to direct patients to the best quality online information. Health information the patient obtains

---

[16] Joosten, E.A.G., DeFuentes-Merillas, L., de Weert, G.H. et al. 2008. Systematic review of the effects of shared decision-making on patient satisfaction, treatment adherence and health status. *Psychotherapy and Psychosomatics*, 77(4), 219–226.

Searching Skills Toolkit: Finding the Evidence, Second Edition. Caroline De Brún and Nicola Pearce-Smith.
© 2014 John Wiley & Sons, Ltd. Published 2014 by John Wiley & Sons, Ltd.

independently from the Internet can be of varying levels of quality, relevance and reliability. This is because the information may have been written using:
- patient or carer experience
- lay person opinion
- drug or pharmaceutical company data
- professional expertise, e.g. GP, nurse, surgeon
- research evidence.

Poor quality health information

People do use the Internet to find out more information about health issues, and 'half of health information searches are on behalf of someone else'.[17] However, in another piece of research, the authors found that only 39% of 500 health websites gave correct information.[18] Many other papers found the same thing, that online health information is of poor quality. So, while patients and carers have access to the Internet and online health information, what they find is not always of the best quality. Many health systems are encouraging patient involvement and shared decision-making. However, to make an informed decision, patients and carers need access to good quality information and this is why health professionals need to know where to look.

Good quality health information

Patients may encounter difficulties when searching the Internet for health information. Material may be written by clinicians, for clinicians, and use language that is not appropriate for the lay person.

Terminology can be problematic, particularly if you are unfamiliar with the alternative names given to conditions; in other countries, for example, ME (myalgic encephalomyelitis) is also known as chronic fatigue syndrome or chronic fatigue immune dysfunction syndrome.

A related issue is the many differences between British and American spelling. If you only search for behaviour with a 'u', you might miss out on important international research, likewise with oestrogen/estrogen, diarrhoea/diarrhea, leukaemia/leukemia and paediatrics/pediatrics.

Awareness of narrower and broader terms is also important. For example, when searching for Crohn's disease, the broader term of inflammatory bowel disease should also be considered.

[17]Fox, S., Duggan, M. 2013 *Health Online 2013*. Pew Research Center, Washington, D.C.

[18]Scullard, P., Peacock, C., Davies, P. 2010 Googling children's health: reliability of medical advice on the Internet. *Archives of Disease in Childhood*, 95(5), 580–582.

Behind the Headlines

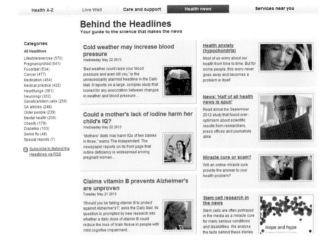

Behind the Headlines
Your guide to the science that makes the news

Categories
All Headlines
Lifestyle/exercise (570)
Pregnancy/child (541)
Food/diet (534)
Cancer (477)
Medication (454)
Medical practice (422)
Heart/lungs (381)
Neurology (352)
Genetics/stem cells (256)
QA articles (248)
Older people (239)
Mental health (206)
Obesity (179)
Diabetes (103)
Swine flu (48)
Special reports (7)

Subscribe to Behind the Headlines via RSS

Cold weather may increase blood pressure
Wednesday May 22 2013

'Bad weather could raise your blood pressure and even kill you,' is the unnecessarily alarmist headline in the Daily Mail. It reports on a large, complex study that looked for any association between changes in weather and blood pressure...

Could a mother's lack of iodine harm her child's IQ?
Wednesday May 22 2013

'Mothers' diets may harm IQs of two babies in three,' warns The Independent. The newspaper reports on its front page that iodine deficiency is widespread among pregnant women...

Claims vitamin B prevents Alzheimer's are unproven
Tuesday May 21 2013

'Should you be taking vitamin B to protect against Alzheimer's?,' asks the Daily Mail. Its question is prompted by new research into whether a daily dose of vitamin B could reduce the loss of brain tissue in people with mild cognitive impairment...

Health anxiety (hypochondria)

Most of us worry about our health from time to time. But for some people, this worry never goes away and becomes a problem in itself

News: 'Half of all health news is spun'

Read about the September 2012 study that found over-optimism about scientific results from researchers, press offices and journalists alike

Miracle cure or scam?

Will an online miracle cure provide the answer to your health problem?

Stem cell research in the news

Stem cells are often portrayed in the media as a miracle cure for many serious conditions and disabilities. We analyse the facts behind these stories

Hope and hype

One resource that is particularly useful is Behind the Headlines www.nhs.uk/news/, a service delivered by NHS Choices. Newspapers often report the benefits of new interventions, promising cure-alls and miracles, but they don't always provide the whole picture. Patients and carers see these articles too and may be convinced that it is the right treatment for them. It is important that they can find all the information and not just the media highlights. Behind the Headlines takes the newspaper article and within 48 hours, identifies and analyses the original research, publishing it in a reader-friendly format, and providing a brief conclusion giving the facts about whether the treatment is beneficial to everyone or not. The service is freely available to all and is useful to both health professionals and patients.

Appraising online consumer health information

Appraising online consumer health information is an important step, particularly if you have found the information by searching an unfiltered Internet search engine such as Google or Yahoo. Fortunately, guidance and supporting tools are available, and these are described in greater depth in Chapter 4: Searching the Internet.

As a quick guide, good quality patient information should have the following features:

- Written clearly for the patient, and describing the risks and benefits involved.
- Easily accessible in a variety of formats including online and hard copy (paper).
- Content based on current and relevant scientific evidence.
- Conflicts of interest should be clearly described.
- Author credentials visible.

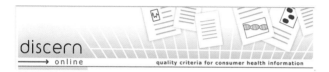

Discern (www.discern.org.uk/)
This is a tool created by the Department of Public Health, University of Oxford, that can help people evaluate the quality of online patient information. It is a checklist which prompts you to think about how the information was created and therefore whether it is high quality or not. It is useful, particularly for rarer conditions, where there might not be very much information available.

Trusted information sources

There are a range of freely-available and trusted health information sources, which make it much easier for people to access patient information:

NHS Choices (www.nhs.uk/)
This site is the main page for NHS users. It provides good quality information about local services and conditions, together with well-being advice, and support networks for a range of patient groups. The National Health Service for England has developed this site as a gateway to quality patient information on common conditions and NHS services. The site also has a feature which translates the information into a range of languages, including Polish, Chinese and Bengali.

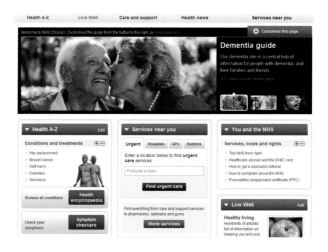

Department of Health Information Standard
(www.theinformationstandard.org/)

The Department of Health Information Standard is awarded to patient information publishers who have met strict criteria relating to the quality of the process and content of the patient information that they are producing. If a website displays the IS logo, it should contain high quality information. This is a certification scheme which helps the public and patients quickly identify reliable sources of quality, evidence-based information. Patient information providers go through a rigorous process at the end of which they are awarded certification, added to a list of high-quality information providers, and are entitled to display a standard on their website and leaflets.

NICE Evidence Search (www.evidence.nhs.uk)
This site is designed by and for clinicians, but it does contain information for patients, which has been assessed for quality. Use the 'Type of Information' navigation button to the left of the results to restrict your search to patient information.

Equip (www.equip.nhs.uk)
This site links to freely-available quality patient information leaflets, translated into many different languages.

Healthfinder.gov (www.healthfinder.gov/HealthTopics/)
This site contains links to patient information on a range of conditions, written predominantly in English and Spanish.

HealthTalk Online (www.healthtalkonline.org/)
HealthTalk Online is a collection of patient experiences covering about 50 conditions. They have been systematically collated by the University of Oxford, and follow a consistent structure.

YouthHealthTalk Online (www.youthhealthtalk.org/)
YouthHealthTalk Online complements HealthTalk Online but focuses on conditions and experiences more relevant to young people.

NHS Direct (www.nhsdirect.nhs.uk/)
This site works closely with NHS Choices. It allows patients to check their symptoms, access good quality patient information, and speak to qualified professionals for advice.

NHS Shared Decision-Making (www.sdm.rightcare.nhs.uk/)
This is a collection of decision aids that enable patients to be more involved in the decisions made about their treatments. It allows you to browse a list of decision aids or search for a condition using keywords. There are currently over 30 decision aids available.

Testing Treatments Interactive (www.testingtreatments.org)
Testing Treatments Interactive is an interactive book aimed at patients and health professionals, to help them understand more about how to differentiate between good and bad research, and to learn more about clinical trials.

As with all online information, it is important to check for whom the information was intended. Different countries may not manage conditions in the same way, so some treatments may not be relevant or appropriate for your patient population. For example, drug dosages may differ between countries.

Rarer conditions

Finding good quality health information on rarer conditions can be much harder, because the higher level of research study (e.g. controlled trials, systematic reviews) are not available. Evidence for rarer conditions is often in the form of case reports and personal experience via support groups. There are some sites which support rarer conditions, but if not, it may be necessary to carry out a search on the Internet, using hints and tips described in Chapter 4: Searching the Internet.

Chapter 4: Searching the Internet

Madisons Foundation (www.madisonsfoundation.org/)
This organisation was set up to help connect parents whose children have the same rare disease, and also to signpost them to medical information. Together with a team of medical specialists, the Foundation has created a library of rare paediatric disease write-ups.

Third-party assistance
Public librarians or hospital-based Patient Advisory Liaison Services may also be able to help patients/carers find good quality health information.

Patient decision aids
Patient decision aids are evidence-based tools which help people make informed choices about their healthcare, while allowing them to maintain their personal values and preferences. Many organisations are developing decision aids, and some key developers include:

NHS Decision-Making Programme
(www.sdm.rightcare.nhs.uk/pda/)
This programme has launched 36 online patient decision aids. Designed and developed by Totally Health, the aids aim to help people think about healthcare decisions using information that has been compiled by the BMJ Group to choose the treatment that best suits their needs. The decision aids include abdominal aortic aneurysm repair, cataracts, established kidney failure, kidney dialysis and kidney transplant, etc.

Ottawa Hospital Research Institute
(www.decisionaid.ohri.ca/AZlist.html)
This is a collection of decision aids organised by health topic.

International Patient Decision Aids Standards (IPDAS)
(www.ipdasi.org/2006%20IPDAS%20Quality%20Checklist.pdf)
This resource provides standards for the development of patient decision aids.

Agency for Healthcare Research and Quality
(www.effectivehealthcare.ahrq.gov/index.cfm/tools-and-resources/
patient-decision-aids/)
These decision aids are designed for patients with certain conditions to help
them think about what is important to them when talking with their
clinician about treatment options.

Writing patient information

There is guidance available for those involved with writing patient
information, and here are some of the key resources available:

NHS Identity (www.nhsidentity.nhs.uk/tools-and-resources/
patient-information)
You will need to use NHS branding so it is essential that you follow the
official guidelines. These are very handy because they contain all the logos
that you need.

The Department of Health Information Standard
(www.theinformationstandard.org/)
The Department of Health Information Standard is a rigorous accreditation
process for patient information providers to go through to demonstrate that
their patient information leaflets have been developed to a high standard.
The website provides guidance on how to write good quality consumer
health information.

Keeping up to date with patient information

A useful forum for keeping up to date with patient information
developments is:

The Patient Information Forum (www.pifonline.org.uk/)
This site is the UK association for professionals that work in the field of
consumer health information, and it supports people who produce or
provide health information either for patients and the public.

Finally, remember to use your local librarian if
you are writing patient information or if you need to
find some for your patient, as they can help with
finding the evidence to validate your patient
information.

Further reading

Da Silva, D. 2012. Helping people share decision making. The Health Foundation, London
✓**Full text:** www.health.org.uk/public/cms/75/76/313/3448/
HelpingPeopleShareDecisionMaking.pdf?realName=rFVU5h.pdf

Dobransky, K. & Hargittai, E. 2012. Inquiring minds acquiring wellness: uses of online and
offline sources for health information. *Health Communication*, 27(4), 331–343
available from: PMID: 21932982

Stacey, D., Bennett, C.L., Barry, M.J., Col, N.F., Eden, K.B., Holmes-Rovner, M.,
Llewellyn-Thomas, H., Lyddiatt, A., Légaré, F. & Thomson, R. 2011. Decision aids for
people facing health treatment or screening decisions. *Cochrane Database of
Systematic Reviews*, Issue 10. Art. No.: CD001431
✓**Full text:** www.onlinelibrary.wiley.com/doi/10.1002/14651858.CD001431.pub3/pdf

Peterson, G., Aslani, P. & Williams, K.A. 2003. How do consumers search for and appraise
information on medicines on the Internet? A qualitative study using focus groups.
Journal of Medical Internet Research, 5(4), e33 available from: PMCID: PMC1550579
✓**Full text:** www.jmir.org/2003/4/e33/

CHAPTER 14
Critical appraisal

The majority of content indexed in healthcare databases has not undergone additional critical appraisal. The Cochrane Library contains systematic reviews that have been conducted in accordance with strict guidelines, but if the information you are looking for is not available in the Cochrane Library, then you will need to search other databases, such as Medline, Embase, CINAHL or PsycINFO. The papers indexed on these databases are not appraised by the indexers, and consequently their quality is variable. This section contains some resources for appraising documents.

Definition
Critical appraisal means being able to look at a paper in an objective and structured way, so that you can be confident about the validity and quality of the paper.

If you are supporting a treatment decision based on a published paper, you want to be sure that the research has been carried out reliably and accurately, with minimum bias. Published papers are not always reliable and may not always be relevant to your patient population. The critical appraisal process should entail a fair assessment of the research, weighing up the strengths and weaknesses, benefits and limitations.

The purpose of critical appraisal is to find out the answers to the following three questions:
1. What are the results?
2. Are the results valid?
3. How will these results help me in my work?

Critical appraisal checklists
There are many checklists and tools available to help support critical appraisal, and some are listed:
- Centre for Evidence-Based Medicine – checklists and tools
  www.cebm.net
- Critical Appraisal Skills Programme (CASP) – tools
  www.casp-uk.net/
- The GATE Frame – tool with pictures
  www.fmhs.auckland.ac.nz/soph/depts/epi/epiq/_docs/gateframe.pdf
- Scottish Intercollegiate Guidelines Network – checklists
  www.sign.ac.uk/methodology/checklists.html

Searching Skills Toolkit: Finding the Evidence, Second Edition. Caroline De Brún and Nicola Pearce-Smith.
© 2014 John Wiley & Sons, Ltd. Published 2014 by John Wiley & Sons, Ltd.

For a brief overview of critical appraisal, download this article from
Bandolier: www.medicine.ox.ac.uk/bandolier/booth/glossary/Critapp.html

See also: Heneghan and Badenoch's (2006) *Evidence-based Medicine
Toolkit*. Part of the *EBMT-EBM Toolkit Series*, this book covers the key
elements of evidence-based medicine, including the critical appraisal of
different types of study.

Many institutions provide training in critical appraisal because it plays such
an important role in evidence-based practice, so it is worth contacting your
local library to see whether they run courses.

Further reading

Akobeng, A.K. 2005. Understanding systematic reviews and meta-analysis. *Arch Dis Child*,
90(8), 845–848 available from: PM:16040886
✓**Full text:** www.adc.bmj.com/content/90/8/845.full

Akobeng, A.K. 2005. Understanding randomised controlled trials. *Arch Dis Child*, 90(8),
840–844 available from: PM:16040885
✓**Full text:** www.adc.bmj.com/content/90/8/840.full

Booth, A. & Brice, A. 2004. Appraising the evidence, In *Evidence based practice for
information professionals: a handbook*, Booth, A. & Brice, A., eds, Facet Publishing,
London, pp. 96–109
✓**Full text:** www.facetpublishing.co.uk/downloads/file/sample_chapters/481.pdf

Greenhalgh, T. 1997. How to read a paper. Papers that report drug trials. *BMJ*,
315(7106), 480–483 available from: PM:9284672
✓**Full text:** www.bmj.com/about-bmj/resources-readers/publications/how-read-paper

Heneghan, C. & Badenoch, D. 2006. *Evidence-based Medicine Toolkit*. 2nd ed. Blackwell
Publishing Ltd., Oxford

Hou, W. & Carden, D. 2012. Statistics for the nonstatistician: Part II. *South Med J*, 105(3),
131–135 available from: PM:22392208

Jackson, R., Ameratunga, S., Broad, J., Connor, J., et al. 2006. The GATE frame: critical
appraisal with pictures. *ACP Journal Club*, 144(2), A8–A11 available from:
PM:17213070
✓**Full text:** www.fmhs.auckland.ac.nz/soph/depts/epi/epiq/_docs/gateframe.pdf

Mansi, I.A. 2012. Statistics for the nonstatistician: A primer for reading clinical studies.
South Med J, 105(3), 120–125 available from: PM:22392206

Timm, D.F., Banks, D.E. & McLarty, J. 2012. Critical appraisal process: step-by-step. *South
Med J*, 105(3), 144–148 available from: PM:22392210

Young, J.M. & Solomon, M.J. 2009. How to critically appraise an article. *Nat Clin Pract
Gastroenterol Hepatol*, 6(2), 82–91 available from: PM:19153565
✓**Full text:** www.nature.com/nrgastro/journal/v6/n2/full/ncpgasthep1331.html

Wissing, D.R. & Timm, D. 2012. Statistics for the nonstatistician: Part I. *South Med J*,
105(3), 126–130 available from: PM:22392207

CHAPTER 15
Glossary of terms

Abstract
This is a short, structured or unstructured summary of the paper, often word limited to about 150 to 300 words. The abstract appears in healthcare databases and at the start of a published paper.

Adjacent (ADJ)
This is also referred to as 'with'. It is useful when searching for phrases which contain smaller connecting words such as of, the, by, for, etc. For example, 'community adj1 practice' will find results containing the phrase 'community of practice'.

Aggregator
This is also known as a feed reader or a news reader and it is an online service which is used for collecting RSS feeds as does Microsoft Outlook. Many web browsers have a facility to collect RSS feeds. Alternatively, NetVibes (www.netvibes.com/en) or Hootsuite (www.hootsuite.com/dashboard) are also available.

AND
This is a Boolean operator which narrows the search results so that all terms are searched for, e.g. venous thrombosis AND compression stockings.

Blogs
This is an example of web 2.0 technology, and is short for Web log. It is an online journal where people can post news, comments and thoughts. Many resources, including journals use blogs to promote new content. Blogger (www.blogger.com) and WordPress (www.wordpress.com) are examples of blog software.

Boolean operators
Boolean operators are words which facilitate the combination of search terms, allowing the search to be limited or widened.

Broader term
This is the opposite of narrowing a search and it means that the search is less specific regarding the search term, thus avoiding the issue of missing out on relevant research.

Searching Skills Toolkit: Finding the Evidence, Second Edition. Caroline De Brún and Nicola Pearce-Smith.
© 2014 John Wiley & Sons, Ltd. Published 2014 by John Wiley & Sons, Ltd.

Browser

This is the software that lets you view the Internet / World Wide Web. Internet Explorer, Safari, Chrome, and Mozilla Firefox are all types of browser.

Citation

This provides all the information that is needed to find the research paper when the full text is not available online. A citation is made up of:
- the title of the paper
- the name(s) of the author(s)
- the source (e.g. journal title, date, volume, part/issue number, page numbers).

Citation index

This is a bibliographic tool which helps track when and where a piece of research has been cited in subsequent pieces of research.

Citation manager

This is a piece of software that stores citations and abstracts retrieved from the search database. They can then be manipulated and used in a format to support document creation, collation of references, etc. Examples of citation managers include:
- Mendeley
  www.mendeley.com
- EndNote
  www.endnote.com/

Citation pearl searching

This is another method of searching for literature. It looks at:
- other papers by the same author(s)
- the references that the authors have used to see what papers those authors looked at
- the keywords that the authors have used in their search strategy
- related similar items – this option is appearing more often in databases.

Clinical Queries

This is a service which was originally developed by PubMed, which built filters into the database, based on those created by the team at McMaster University. There are two types of filtered search available:

1. Question type – this search finds citations that correspond to a specific clinical study category, e.g. aetiology, diagnosis, therapy, prognosis, or clinical prediction guides. There is also the option to create a narrow, specific search or a broad, sensitive search.

2. Systematic reviews – this search finds citations for systematic reviews, meta-analyses, reviews of clinical trials, evidence-based medicine, consensus development conferences, and guidelines.

Clinical Queries is available here: www.ncbi.nlm.nih.gov/pubmed/clinical

Combining

This activity helps to build an effective search strategy because it joins the terms together, using Boolean operators, so that relevant results are retrieved.

Commissioning

Commissioning enables health services to operate more effectively and efficiently by making informed decisions based on assessment of needs, and evidence about purchasing and resource allocation.

Controlled vocabulary

This is also known as MeSH, index terms, keywords; they are a few words which identify the content of the research, and they are added to the thesaurus or index.

Cost-effectiveness analysis

This highlights treatment interventions which are relatively low in cost, yet make substantial improvements to the outcome of the patient.

Critical appraisal

Systematic assessment of the methods that have been applied to carry out the research, to ensure that it has been written to high standards, is reliable and trustworthy. Checklists to facilitate this process are available here: www.casp-uk.net/

Database

This is a searchable computer system which stores and indexes all the abstracts from the research. Examples include PubMed/Medline, CINAHL, PsycINFO, HMIC and Embase.

Descriptors

Also known as MeSH, subject headings, index terms, etc. these are keywords that have been assigned to each article and added to a thesaurus and index.

Email alerts

Many resources provide a service which lets users know when new content has been added or new articles have been published. The results are sent via email.

Explode term
This concept is part of the thesaurus feature, and enables the search to be extended to include narrower terms.

Feed reader
This is also known as an aggregator or a news reader and it is an online service which is used for collecting RSS feeds as does Microsoft Outlook. Many web browsers have a facility to collect RSS feeds. Alternatively, Google Reader (www.google.com/reader), NetVibes (www.netvibes.com/en) or Hootsuite (www.hootsuite.com/dashboard) are also available.

Filter
McMaster University has developed a set of search strategies, which direct the database to find research of a particular publication type. By applying one of these filters, for example the filter for systematic reviews, to a search, the database will find all systematic reviews which match the search terms entered. PubMed was the first to offer this feature in the form of 'Clinical Queries', but now many other databases are incorporating filters.

Focus
This feature means that the database will search for the term as a major subheading, e.g. any records found will have the term describing an important aspect of the article.

Free text
The words are typed into the database as they would be spoken or spelled.

History
This feature appears on most databases and is a record of all the searches carried out during a particular search session.

Hyperlinks
These are electronic connections which take you to another page or somewhere else in the document.

Index terms
Also known as MeSH, subject headings, index terms, etc. these are keywords that have been assigned to each article and added to a thesaurus and index.

Information
This is facts, knowledge or concepts which have been received or communicated.

Information literacy
This is the ability to identify an information need, find the information, and appraise the quality and reliability of it.

Internet
This is also known as the World Wide Web, and is a vast collection of knowledge and information on all topics, created by a range of authors, both expert and non-expert.

Keywords
These are also known as controlled vocabulary, MeSH, descriptors and index terms; they are a few words which identify the content of the research, and they are added to the thesaurus or index.

Knowledge
This is acquired on an individual basis, as a result of interaction and learning. It is also known as wisdom, expertise, intuition, etc.

Level of evidence
This is a hierarchy of study designs according to their internal validity, or degree to which they are not susceptible to bias. They are available at www.cebm.net/index.aspx?o=1025

Limit
Databases have varying limit options. Some have very comprehensive options, for example Medline, which allows the age to be broken up into 13 stages of life, including newborn, middle-aged, and aged. Limit options include language, publication type, gender etc.

MeSH
This stands for Medical Subject Headings. Also known as MeSH, subject headings, index terms, etc. these are keywords that have been assigned to each article and added to a thesaurus and index.

Narrower term
This is a word which is much more specific, allowing the search to be more focused. For example, rather than searching for 'nurse' a narrower term might be 'community nurse'.

Natural language
The words are typed into the database as they would be spoken, without being refined.

NEAR
This is used as a Boolean operator and it means that all the words will be searched in a specific order, for example as a phrase.

NOT
This is used as a Boolean operator and it means that only one of the terms will be searched for, for example 'contraception' NOT 'oral' would exclude research on oral contraceptives.

Open access
This refers to research which is freely accessible to all via the World Wide Web. Biomed Central (www.biomedcentral.com/) is an example of a supplier of online open access journals.

Open source
This refers to computer programs where the source code has been made freely available by the authors, so that it can be developed by other authors to create new programs. Linux (www.linux.org) is an example of the open source initiative.

OR
This is used as a Boolean operator and it means that the database will search for one or other of the terms, or for research containing both terms.

PICO
This is the acronym for a framework for building focused, clinical questions. The 'P' represents the patient, problem or population; the 'I' stands for intervention, for example the treatment; 'C' is for comparison (optional); 'O' stands for outcome.

Primary research
This refers to original studies such as a randomised controlled trial, cohort study etc., where data are collected from experiments, observation, and case studies.

Publication type
This describes the format of publication, for example it may be a journal article, a letter, an editorial, a book or a report.

Qualitative data
Research in which the data are numerical and which seeks to test hypotheses by statistical analysis of the data.

Quantitative data
Analysis and identification of concepts and common themes. The research is based on opinions and statements, as opposed to statistics.

Randomised Controlled Trials (RCTs)
Are a particular type of study which tests the effectiveness of treatments within a specific patient population who have been randomly allocated to the treatment. The following are recommended sources for finding RCTs.

Respected authorities
These refer to societies, associations, Royal colleges, etc. which inform and influence the development and activities of the professions they represent.

RSS feeds 🔊
This is web 2.0 software and is available on many sites. It is a method for being notified of new content on websites or newly-published research in journals. RSS feeds are recognisable by an orange button, either with XML, RSS or a symbol on it, as shown. An aggregator/feed reader is required to collect the RSS feeds. A useful tutorial on RSS is available from Common Craft. The video called 'RSS in Plain English' is available at www.commoncraft.com/rss_plain_english

Search engines
Online tools to navigate the Internet, search for information, and retrieve relevant web pages. Examples include Google (www.google.co.uk) and Yahoo (www.yahoo.co.uk).

Search strategy
A combination of search terms identified from a focused clinical question which, when entered into a database, aim to retrieve relevant papers.

Secondary research
A summary or synthesis of existing primary research, for example a systematic review.

Secondary sources
Secondary sources of information contain reviews of primary research. Sources could include a summary of the literature in a scientific paper published in a journal, an overview of a disease or treatment in a book, or a synthesis written to review the available literature on a topic.

Sensitivity
In searching, sensitivity is high recall, low precision, in other words more of the relevant articles are retrieved but at the expense of picking up more unwanted articles.

Single citation matcher
This is a service provided by PubMed which helps locate the full reference of a research paper, when only partial information is available. Single citation manager is available here: www.ncbi.nlm.nih.gov/pubmed/citmatch

Snowballing
This is an enhanced searching technique, where you follow up the references in one paper to identify other papers which are relevant for your research, but which may not have been captured in the literature search.

Social bookmarking
This is web 2.0 software and allows users to store bookmarks online so that they are accessible from any computer. The bookmarks can also be shared with colleagues, and can be catalogued or tagged by adding keywords. Diigo (www.diigo.com/) is an example of a social bookmarking tool.

Specificity
In searching, specificity is lower recall, higher precision, in other words more of the articles retrieved will be relevant (proportionally), but some of the relevant articles may be missed.

Subheadings
Subheadings appear as an option in the index terms of most healthcare databases. MeSH, for example, will allow you to select from a range of subheadings. It allows you to refine/focus your search even further, by selecting one or more subheadings from a range of choices.

Summary
This is a shortened version of a document, for example a synopsis, providing the key points.

Synonyms
These are alternative terms meaning the same thing and are useful for comprehensive searching, e.g. venous thrombosis and deep vein thrombosis.

Text word
Healthcare databases search for free text words in the title or abstract of the document.

Thesaurus
Also known as controlled vocabulary, subject headings, index terms, etc. these are keywords that have been assigned to each article and added to a thesaurus and index.

Truncation

Truncation can be used to pick up different word endings in a search. It is usually a * or $ symbol, and acts as a substitute for any string of zero or more characters at the end of a word. For example, the search aggress* retrieves aggression, aggressive, aggressor etc.

Uniform Resource Locators (URLs)

This is the address of a website, most commonly starting with 'http' (hypertext transfer protocol).

Web 2.0

This is the second generation of the Internet and provides tools which enable people to keep up to date with information, share knowledge, and work together. Examples of web 2.0 technology include RSS, blogs, social bookmarking, wikis.

Wikis

Wikis are online spaces where groups of people can edit documents together. They are useful for people working on the same project but who are geographically spread. An example of wiki software is Wikispaces (www.wikispaces.com).

Wildcard

A wildcard can be used to represent one or more characters. It can be used to include British English or American English spelling, or sometimes to include both singular and plural words. A wildcard symbol is usually a question mark. For example, 'behavio?r' or 'wom?n'.

World Wide Web (WWW)

The World Wide Web, also known as the Internet, is a collection of knowledge and information on all topics, created by a range of authors, both expert and non-expert.

APPENDIX 1

Ten tips for effective searching

1. Turn the clinical problem into a searchable question and pull out the keywords. The PICO framework is a good template to use as it enables you to be clear in the outcomes:
   Scenario: A GP wants to know whether mobile phones put children at risk of leukaemia and other cancers.

Patient Problem Population	Intervention/Exposure	Outcome
Children	Mobile phone calls	Leukaemia
Infants	Smart phone calls	Leukemia
Preschool	Cell phone calls	Cancer
Toddlers	Cellular phone calls	Neoplasms
Adolescents		Brain cancer
	Comparison	
	Text messaging	

2. Make a list of alternative terms that might be used for each of the key concepts; never rely on any one term as you may miss out on relevant research! For example, searching for the term 'mobile phones' may miss out many relevant articles if you do not also search for 'cell phone' or 'cellular'.
3. When searching databases, search one database at a time and search for one term at a time. If you search for all terms at once and you find no results, you will need to start all over again, while if you have searched for them separately, you can form different combinations of terms until you get the results that you need.
4. There are two ways of searching databases. For best results, start with a thesaurus search and combine with a free text search:
   • Thesaurus (also known as MeSH or subject heading) searches – every article that is added to the databases is also tagged with a set of index terms, and these form the thesaurus. By searching for terms in the thesaurus, only papers that are specifically about that subject, and similar terms, will be retrieved, so the results will be much more relevant. However, it takes time for the articles to be indexed, or

Searching Skills Toolkit: Finding the Evidence, Second Edition. Caroline De Brún and Nicola Pearce-Smith.
© 2014 John Wiley & Sons, Ltd. Published 2014 by John Wiley & Sons, Ltd.

sometimes, if it is a new intervention, there may not be an index term yet, and so it is important to combine thesaurus searches with free text.
- Free text (also known as natural language or keyword) searches – means that the database will search the whole text for the term that you have entered and no others. So it won't look for similar terms, plurals, or spelling variations. Truncation (* or $) and wildcards (?) help to improve retrieval by expanding options, e.g. nurs* will look for nurse, nurses, nursing, while leuk?emia will retrieve papers containing the British spelling for leukaemia and the American spelling (leukemia), saving a little time.

5. Find additional or related search terms from retrieved records:
   - Free text terms in the abstracts and/or titles that have not been included, but should be
   - Thesaurus terms that have not been included, but should be
   - References at the end of the paper.

6. Combine free text and thesaurus search terms under each concept using OR. Then, combine the results of each concept with AND so that you find papers with all the concept terms, and answering your original search question.

7. If too many records are retrieved, go back over the strategy and narrow the search:
   - Use more specific or most relevant terms in free text.
   - Use thesaurus search rather than free text.
   - Use more specific or relevant Thesaurus terms.
   - Select specific subheadings with Thesaurus terms.
   - Add terms for other aspects of question (e.g. age or gender of patient), using AND.
   - Use limits.

8. If too few records retrieved, go back over strategy and widen search:
   - Use more terms: synonyms, related terms, broader terms.
   - Add in terms of related meaning with OR.
   - Combine results of Thesaurus and Free Text searches.
   - Use Explode feature of Thesaurus, which will include narrower terms.
   - Select All Subheadings when searching for Thesaurus terms.

9. Limit search results at the end of the search by:
   - language of article
   - date
   - publication type: e.g. randomised controlled trials, meta-analysis, reviews
   - age.

10. Save search with the name of the database and the date searched, for future reference. You can also set up an alert so that each time another

paper is added to the database that matches your search criteria, then you will automatically be informed. This is a useful way to keep up to date in your field of interest.

Seek support from your local library if you need further assistance, or make use of the help pages in your chosen information source.

Teaching resources

This section includes some ideas for teaching the concepts of search skills to health professionals.

Icebreaker – Imagine you are looking for a restaurant

At the start of a search skills session, show a picture of some food or something you might want to buy, such as a stereo system, and say, 'imagine you are looking for a restaurant, where would you look for choices?' Ask participants to shout out some ideas and write them on a flip chart. Answers might be Yellow Pages, friends, adverts, critic reviews, Internet, television programmes, etc. Explain that you would use the same principles for finding the answers to clinical questions, for example asking colleagues, reading books and articles, Internet, databases, etc. This helps them realise that they are not learning something new and complex. It is something they already do in their daily lives.

Name that database

There are many databases available, which cover health-related topics and it can be quite confusing. This exercise gives the participants a list of the databases available, together with a brief description, including details of content and period of cover. Divide the participants into groups and give them a list of scenarios or clinical questions. Ask them to work within their groups to choose the most suitable database(s) for answering the scenarios or clinical questions. This can also be used to identify which database is most suitable for different types of question, for example prognosis, therapy or diagnosis. The scenarios can then be used in the hands-on search session. Some examples of questions include:

1. What are the benefits of modern matrons? (*HMIC, CINAHL*)
2. Should newborns be vaccinated against chicken pox if the mother has been exposed to the illness? (*Medline/Pubmed, Embase, CINAHL*)
3. Are there any articles about the effects of Prozac on someone suffering from depression? (*Cochrane Library, Embase, Medline/Pubmed*)
4. What adverse drug interactions could arise when treating obesity with alternative medicines, in a patient with heart disease? (*AMED, Medline/ Pubmed, Embase*)

Searching Skills Toolkit: Finding the Evidence, Second Edition. Caroline De Brún and Nicola Pearce-Smith.
© 2014 John Wiley & Sons, Ltd. Published 2014 by John Wiley & Sons, Ltd.

5. What sources are most reliable for identifying examples of quality improvement? (*Cochrane Effective Practice and Organisation of Care Group, PDQ-Evidence, TRIP Database*)

Terminology mix and match

The aim of the glossary exercise is to familiarise people with the terminology used in searching, critical appraisal, and research. You prepare one set of cards with the terms on them and another set with the definitions. You mix them all up and the participants have to work together to match the pairs. You can have more than one set of cards depending on how big the group is. It is a useful exercise because it provokes discussion and helps people to remember what the terms mean. Terms will differ depending on what is being taught.

Examples of cards:

Systematic review	A review of a clearly formulated question that uses systematic and explicit methods to identify, select and critically appraise relevant research, and to collect and analyse data from the studies that are included in the review
Text word	Free text fields refer to those words that have not been individually indexed in the database
Thesaurus	lso known as controlled vocabulary, subject headings, index terms, etc. these are keywords that have been assigned to each article and added to a thesaurus and index
Truncation	This symbol (often * or $) can be used when searching. The symbol acts as a substitute for any string of zero or more characters at the end of a word. For example, the search aggress* retrieves aggression, aggressive, aggressor
Qualitative Research	Analysis and identification of concepts and common themes. The research is based on opinions and statements, as opposed to statistics
Quantitative Research	Research in which the data are numerical and which seeks to test hypotheses by statistical analysis of the data

Create more cards using the terms listed in the glossary of this book.

Comparing different sources of information

An effective icebreaker for larger groups is to split them up and allocate three types of information source to each group, for example Medline, colleagues and books for one group and Cochrane Library, Internet and journals for the second group. An example to give to the groups is 'newspapers'. Give them about 10 minutes to discuss and list, within their groups, the advantages and disadvantages of their assigned information sources.

After 10 minutes, ask each group to feed back to the group as a whole, inviting brief comments. This exercise helps people to understand why you need to think about which are the best sources of information for people to use when searching for quality health information. Answers might include:

Information Source	Advantages	Disadvantages
Book	• easy to access • greater depth of coverage than journals • overview of subject • portable • reduced cost – borrow from library • good reference	• quickly out of date • quality of indexing varies • time consuming to search/scan • expensive • access to libraries may be limited • author/publisher bias
Internet	• up-to-date • valuable/unique information • etc.	• no central directory • information and sites are difficult to locate • etc.
Journals	• current • may be peer reviewed (integrity) • etc.	• time-consuming to search/scan • expensive • etc.
Etc.		

Search off

This exercise is useful for familiarising participants with the electronic evidence resources available to them, giving them the confidence to search by letting them explore in a safe environment with expertise on hand to help.

First of all identify a relevant scenario, formulate a question, and create a PICO framework. Describe a range of resources, such as the TRIP database, NICE Evidence Search, Google Scholar, PubMed Clinical Queries, PubMed, UpToDate, Clinical Evidence, DynaMed, Cochrane Library etc., briefly outlining the differences between each resource.

Allocate these resources so that each person has at least one to search, and then ask them to find the answer to the question using the terms generated from the PICO framework. Suggest that they note down how many results they retrieve and what terms they used. If they find the answer quickly, then encourage them to try some of the other resources, and compare the results.

After 10 minutes, bring everyone back to the group and ask them to share their experiences, describing what worked and what didn't work for them. Record the responses on a PowerPoint slide so that the group has an aide-memoire for the future.

It is useful to prepare some handouts with the instructions, scenario, empty PICO framework, names and URLs of the resources, and a table to note down results for reporting back.

Record your favourite resources

If you have any suggestions for improving this toolkit, or if you think that a useful resource is missing from this toolkit, please contact the publisher, so that the next edition can be improved.

Searching Skills Toolkit: Finding the Evidence, Second Edition. Caroline De Brún and Nicola Pearce-Smith.
© 2014 John Wiley & Sons, Ltd. Published 2014 by John Wiley & Sons, Ltd.

Index

Page numbers in *italics* denote figures, those in **bold** denote tables.

Searching Skills Toolkit: Finding the Evidence, Second Edition. Caroline De Brún and
Nicola Pearce-Smith.
© 2014 John Wiley & Sons, Ltd. Published 2014 by John Wiley & Sons, Ltd.